# EXPERIENCES OF HYSTERECTOMY

## ANN WEBB

An OPTIMA book

First published in 1989 by
Macdonald Optima, a division of
Macdonald & Co. (Publishers) Ltd

A member of Maxwell Pergamon Publishing Corporation plc

British Library Cataloguing in Publication Data

Webb, Ann
    Experiences of hysterectomy.
    1. Women. Uterus. Hysterectomy
    I. Title
    618.1′453

    ISBN 0-356-14141-1


Macdonald & Co (Publishers) Ltd
66-73 Shoe Lane
London EC4P 4AB

Typeset in Century Schoolbook
by Leaper & Gard Ltd, Bristol, England

Made and printed in Great Britain by
The Guernsey Press Co. Ltd., Guernsey, Channel Islands.

To Nola Ishmael, who said 'Go for it'.

# ACKNOWLEDGMENTS

I would like to thank the Hysterectomy Support Group and the many women there who have not only contributed to the book, but have also encouraged and supported me. Additional thank yous to Sally Haslett; the librarians at Lewisham Hospital Medical Library; and to my husband Peter and my children.

# CONTENTS

# 1.
# INTRODUCTION

Feelings about hysterectomy can vary a great deal and yet few books take a close look at these from the woman's point of view. The following pages take an in-depth look at women's emotions from the moment they hear the word hysterectomy to a point in time after surgery has been done. This chapter looks first at common thoughts about the operation, starting with what is hysterectomy and what is its place in our lives today?

Confusion can arise about hysterectomy because of the different terms used. In *sub-total* hysterectomy only the womb is removed leaving the cervix or mouth of the womb at the top of the vagina. This used to be common practice, but today a *total* hysterectomy with removal of womb *and* cervix is usual. Some gynaecologists leave the cervix, when possible, believing that this is an aid to sexual sensation and pleasure for the woman. Keeping the cervix means a monthly staining can occur at period times and cervical smears will still be necessary. Total hysterectomy is sometimes thought to mean the ovaries and Fallopian tubes have been removed, but this is not so. The term for this is salpingo (tube)-oophorectomy (ovary) and if both are removed with the womb it would be a total hysterectomy with bilateral (both sides) salpingo-oophorectomy. Often it's simpler for women to say 'the lot has been taken away'. In some cases of extensive pelvic disease, for instance, cancer, a *radical* or Wertheim's hysterectomy may be performed. This involves the removal of the womb, cervix, lymph glands, top third of the vagina, fatty tissue and sometimes the tubes and ovaries. It may also involve treatment with radium.

There are two possible routes for hysterectomy, the most common being through a cut in the abdomen, abdominal hysterectomy. The other is through the vagina, when there is no abdominal cut, vaginal hysterectomy. In the latter, recovery is usually quicker as the abdominal muscles have not been involved. Vaginal hysterectomy is more likely when prolapse is present and/or the womb is not greatly enlarged. The vagina is left intact in both.

Although hysterectomy (vaginal) for prolapse was recorded as long ago as the seventh century AD, hysterectomy in any form was not normal practice until the 1900s. Before this, surgeons operated quickly and on superficial levels of the body without anaesthetic. Excision of the womb was performed only for very serious cases such as cancer, and usually the patient died. The expertise of surgeon and increased survival of patient came with the discovery and improved use of general anaesthetics in the nineteenth century. Even then in the early days of use, there were few survivors of hysterectomy and it was used as a desperate attempt to save life. Eugene Koebolic is seen as the pioneer of hysterectomy. Efficient and safe hysterectomies are improvements of the twentieth century. The operation has developed from being a clumsy attempt to save life to a smooth, simple, surgical technique for the gynaecologist, who may do hundreds in the course of his career. Various estimates put the present number of hysterectomies a year in the UK between 60,000 and 80,000.

For the woman it is still a one-off experience and major surgery. Some wonder if it really is necessary, not realizing that hysterectomy can be classified in three different ways. Prophylactive (preventative) hysterectomy removes a healthy organ considered useless and a possible source of infection and disease. This is rarely done in the UK. Elective hysterectomy is most common, performed when non-life-threatening conditions lower the quality of life, and affect the woman's ability to function as she wishes. Some delay or alternative treatments may be possible. Lastly, non-elective hysterectomy is performed when it is a matter of life or death, either because the patient has cancer or in an emergency situation. Most hysterectomies in the UK are elective and are seen to be an acceptable attempt to improve the quality of life, not only of the woman, but of her family too.

The most longstanding myth seems to be one that is rooted in the name hysterectomy: the fear that problems in the woman's pelvic area may overnight change her into an unreasonable, neurotic person! Worse, that hysterectomy will guarantee a weeping, hysterical, sexless woman about the house and by far the best thing is to ignore her! Hysteria-ectomy would be a suitable name for the fear that many women, and men, have concerning the reasons for, and the effects of, the operation. It all started long ago with Hippocrates, the Father of Medicine. He described a condition called 'hysteria', which followed displacement of the womb towards the liver. Treatment was a simple instruction: If old enough and single, get married; if married or widowed then get pregnant – a familiar piece of advice to some women today, over a thousand years later! Celsus generally considered the greatest Roman medical writer, referred to hysteria as a violent malady arising from the womb, but being different from epilepsy. Aretaeus, the Cappadocian, also viewed hysteria as the result of upper displacement of the womb. Little was known about the diseases that women suffered.

Belief in the hysteria theory was strong in the eighteenth century when excision of the womb became known as hysterectomy. Fortunately this has changed as knowledge about a whole range of body functions and malfunctions has increased. Also earlier strong links to hysteria have lessened as women have progressed from being financially dependent vassals, to individuals with property-owning rights and franchise. Suggestions that hysterectomy was used to control women have faded, as has opposition from the Church. The use of anaesthetic was once seen as Devil-inspired and hysterectomy as a sin against God's commandment to go forth and multiply. But shades of religious or social stricture still remain. Women are only valued, and value themselves, as useful members of society or sexual beings if able to produce a child.

Sometimes women's doubts and fears about hysterectomy seem to be rooted in these misconceptions.Fortunately the concept of hysterectomy is changing and with this people's attitudes. Continuing progress and change in research and patient/doctor relationships give a more positive picture. More doctors are giving women full information and time to discuss hysterectomy. Women, too, are seeking information to enable informed consent to surgery and to allow planning for the recovery period.

Other misconceptions concern the appropriate age for hysterectomy. Most women are ignorant of how their bodies work and what treatments are 'usual' when things go wrong. Many know nothing about hysterectomy or the reasons for it and are shocked when advised that they should have one. Surely, it is something that happens to older, younger, single, married women, or those who've had lots of children, or childless women? In fact, to anyone else but themselves? An 85-year-old spinster, after a vaginal hysterectomy and repair for prolapse, felt 'these things happened to younger women, who'd had lots of babies'. A 40-year-old, due to have a hysterectomy for monthly flooding, had thought the change (menopause) 'just round the corner would solve those sort of problems' and that hysterectomy was for much younger women. A 32-year-old with chronic pelvic inflammatory disease, advised that her ovaries would probably be removed at hysterectomy, felt she was far too young to be having any such operation. An even younger woman, 25 years old, whose hysterectomy for cervical cancer undoubtedly saved her life, had thought it was for 'old women past the change'. Another, aged 19 years, who required an emergency hysterectomy, had never heard of it before.

Shock about the need for a hysterectomy is often accompanied by feelings of isolation, guilt, fear, anger, anxiety and grief.

ISOLATION. Despite the thousands of hysterectomies performed each year, it's not easy to get information in everyday language and this gives rise to feelings of isolation. To question the doctor can be awkward for various reasons and sadly is sometimes seen as the sign of a difficult patient. It's hard to link up with someone in the same sort of situation; socially it's 'not nice' or the 'done thing' to discuss these women's problems.

GUILT. Concern about the impending operation can turn to guilt as medical advisers and perhaps family try to reassure with phrases like 'It's such a common operation, why hesitate?' or 'It's simple, like having your tonsils out. You'll be a new woman!' Guilt can arise at taking time out from work and/or caring for dependents, or simply at being poorly and needing treatment at all. Recovery is hard work, hysterectomy is major surgery no matter how common a procedure it may be. If given unrealistic expectations of recovery, women feel incompetent and inadequate when these aren't matched. They feel guilty when unable to resume full activities immediately on discharge from hospital or at the magical six-week stage.

FEAR is frequently felt of the anaesthetic, the hospital stay, the tubes, bottles and drains connected with surgery; or, fear of being dependent, even for only a few weeks, on someone else. Women may fear that hysterectomy could leave them sexless, fat, prematurely old, frumpy, perpetually depressed, hairy, unfeminine, badly scarred or even a cripple.

ANGER may be felt because there isn't time to be ill, or that a blameless and good healthy life has led to this; that the longed-for baby will never be, or that there won't be another baby. Anger perhaps that some event in the past could so easily have changed the need for surgery, but was overlooked or delayed; or that it just isn't fair.

ANXIETY can arise about domestic arrangements, money, care of dependents, the effect on a partner, children, sex life, and often whether a job will be secure.

GRIEF is felt at the loss of this part of the body that means so much in an emotional context. Loss of the choice to have a baby, of the expected role and path that their life was to have taken. Loss of self-concept and perceived femininity. Or grief submerged from a previous bereavement, merging with the sadness of hysterectomy, to come to the surface and need to be resolved.

For many the actual hysterectomy is less of a worry than the associated treatments and hospital stay. But for most, worry will be replaced by pleasure at the treatment of troublesome symptoms, or of cancer, and by improved health.

Adjustment to the idea of hysterectomy takes time and some seek out information and follow up all sorts of ideas in order to avoid surgery. Others will have been waiting for the opportunity to resolve health problems in this way for years. A number will shy away from details and hope, or be content that the consultant decides on their behalf.

This book looks at the emotional aspect of hysterectomy through the eyes of forty-two women, by following their thoughts and feelings about the whole experience, and how it affects them and their family. As hysterectomy doesn't happen in isolation from other circumstances of life, some of which have a bearing on how women cope, crucial background information is given. Age, marital status, if childless, previous gynaecological resumé and how long ago the operation was performed are details included, where possible, for each woman. Some women had several gynaecological disorders present at the same time. Others had a number of general health problems including asthma, diabetes, long-term depression, or recurrent breast lumps. What becomes apparent is that hysterectomy 'happens' to all types of women, including those with disabilities such as blindness, deafness or physical handicap.

There are different reasons for the operation, but though the chapters are labelled by diagnosis there is only a superficial description of these. There is no in-depth discussion of alternative treatment or social issues involved, other than that which appears as comment by the women in their individual accounts. Many have the same diagnosis but different circumstances and different reactions. Some have different diagnosis but the same reactions. For some it was a catastrophe, for some a mere hiccup, but most feel it would have been helpful to have had more information. They would have liked to have known how others felt and to have had the support that shared experiences can bring.

Selection for inclusion in the book was not random, but based on diagnosis and the numbers needed for each chapter. Quite a few women, but not all, came from the Hysterectomy Support Group and are heavily involved in that voluntary group, as I am. My experience of dealing with the thousands of enquiries to HSG over the past eight years, leads me to feel that the resultant accounts cover the wide spectrum of normality. The two extremes of normality may seem quite opposite, but I would argue that they are valid views and that there isn't a right or a wrong way to feel at any specific time. Nothing should be judged in isolation. I have been, and still am, very moved by the following accounts. I have felt especially privileged to share with each woman her generosity of spirit and the hope that these accounts, this book, may help and support others.

# 2.
# HEAVY, PAINFUL, IRREGULAR BLEEDING

Menorrhagia is the medical word most often used to describe heavy/irregular periods, which may be accompanied by pain at different times of the cycle. The hormones secreted by the ovary – oestrogen and progestogen – react upon the lining of the womb to produce the monthly period. Excessive bleeding may occur if there is a hormonal imbalance or it can be an indication of other disorders, like fibroids or prolapse or pelvic inflammatory disease (PID). Most hysterectomies are performed for menorrhagia and the womb may be called 'bulky' and be tender/painful on examination.

Menorrhagia describes the condition, but not the cause which isn't always found. The laboratory report on the removed womb often comes back with a 'nothing abnormal discovered' tag and the woman is told her womb was healthy. Sometimes women feel this means that the hysterectomy was not needed, but it is simply stating that the cause of the irregularity was not within the womb. Removal of the womb stops the bleeds and usually improves the quality of life experienced by the woman.

All of the six women in this chapter have a different experience of bleeding irregularities. Five have children, one is childless and the ages range from 29 to 50.

## MILLIE

Millie, married for the second time, and with one child, had a total abdominal hysterectomy and ovary removed at

39, a year ago. Her problems began after she had her baby at 16. Her parents refused to allow her to marry the father, but gave her and the baby a home.

'I had bad periods with heavy bleeding and pain, for the next five years. I was sent to hospital for an operation, a small repair job on an ovary. At 22 I married John but we were unsuccessful in starting a family. For seven years I went for infertility tests and treatment. This depressed me, one disappointment after another. Then they discovered I'd only got half an ovary left. One ovary and half of the other had been removed at the 'repair job' all those years earlier. There was no way that I would have any children! It was difficult to come to terms with . . . Why me? Then I found a lump in my breast that needed treatment and an abscess in the other breast led to emergency surgery. The fertility problems got pushed to one side. I began to accept that life wasn't going to give me what I wanted. My marriage broke up after thirteen years; it was a terrible time, and I took an overdose.

'A couple of years later, I met and married Barry, also a divorcee. My health was really bad, tablets weren't helping and I'd had enough, it was getting me down. I paid to see a consultant quickly, and had a D and C (dilation and curettage). It revealed that I needed a hysterectomy, which didn't surprise me. I knew deep down I couldn't go on like I had. It was a relief that something was being done after so much (two years) messing about with "tablets that may help". I feel that family doctors should refer you to someone who knows their job in "special fields". So much time is wasted, and pain suffered, trying different medicines to no avail and the situation gets worse.

'My son, a hospital porter, brought me books from work and told me a lot about the hysterectomy. I work in a library and got a good book out. Even so you can't visualize a picture of yourself being ill until it happens. I was worried about after effects and had the same question as before: "Why me? I'm only 39." Life, I seem to find, has so many questions and not enough answers.

'The National Health Service waiting list was two years. How could I face this? Barry and I talked about it and decided to pay (I wasn't insured) and get it done once and for all. I went into hospital with a brave smile. I had an epidural anaesthetic in the back which really frightened me; I was paralyzed from the chest down for four days. I wondered if I'd ever walk again. Post-op I had every instrument possible – draining tubes, pipes and drips. Slowly each day got better. The consultant had removed the half an ovary as it was in such a mess. I was sent home on the sixth day, which was much too quick. I wondered if I'd ever be well, but each day was better. My bowels were a problem for a month and I got something from the chemist to help. My GP never came near me. I had nine weeks off work and lost a stone in weight. I was glad to get it all over with.

'It is now a year later and I still get very tired and feel no energy. I find eating a full meal weighs on the scar and hurts. I have backache now which I didn't have before. I have Hormone Replacement Therapy (HRT) in an implant, which is renewed every six months. I have to pay for this as my GP refuses to refer me to the NHS. When looking at myself in the bath, I think I should be a woman, look at me I'm like an A to Z map! How much woman is there left of me? The sex side has come off the worst as I have very little interest now. I love Barry very much, but I want him just to hold me in his arms so I feel secure. That's as far as I want it to go. He gets very annoyed, which he's entitled to do, but I don't have any sort of feeling now towards sex. The thought of it just makes me feel "*Oh No!*" In books I've read about hysterectomy it doesn't deal with anything like this, it just says in time sex will resume as before. I hope so.

'The thought of not having the family I wanted doesn't worry me and Barry has two children, now grown up, from his first marriage. He'd also had a vasectomy, so it doesn't make any difference to us.

'I still need treatment for multiple cysts and warts in my breasts. Now that *really* worries me!'

## ANN

Ann, married with one child, had her total abdominal hysterectomy at 42, two months ago.

'I'd experienced severe pain with uncontrollable bleeding for nineteen months. I was fed up with swallowing analgesics and hormone pills. I was positive about the idea of the operation, things could only get better, but when told I needed a hysterectomy my initial feeling was one of fear. I had experienced a disastrous emergency Lower Segment Caesarean Section (LSCS) and post-operation period. I was very frightened. How could I take so much time away from work and from my husband and 19-year-old daughter? How would they cope? How would I cope away from them? How would I manage the initial post-op period, particularly pain control and urinary tract (UTI) problems, which I have suffered with for years? The doctor spent time trying to allay my fears, answering all my questions honestly, but I felt that I had to put up with the symptoms. She asked me to talk to my husband and GP and let her know then. My GP spent ages talking over the pros and cons. My husband was most definitely for the hysterectomy. I think he was suffering as much as myself. So I went ahead.

'It was a shock on the first post-op day to be told by the consultant that I'd had adhesions. These were from the old scar of the LSCS, now removed and re-fashioned, and had pulled the uterus towards the pelvic floor and attached it to my bladder. He had not envisaged the severity of the adhesions or the extent of bladder involvement. I had a six-inch vertical scar on my abdomen.

'Post-op wasn't as bad as I thought it would be. Compared to an emergency LSCS, it was a walkover. Pain control was satisfactory, but I didn't feel in control of myself. After twenty-four hours I asked for oral analgesics which were practically ineffective, but at least I was in control and not in oblivion! Once the intra-venus (IV) line and catheter were removed and I was mobile, I felt much better. The specimen taken before the catheter was removed, showed a urine infection, but as I hadn't complained of any symptoms, they decided not to treat it! A couple of days later I asked for treatment, as I thought I had a UTI, and was then told about the catheter specimen result. The infection proved to be resistant to the first medication and I had the most frightful allergic reaction to the next lot of pills. I was very ill until the next morning, needing an IV infusion and drugs to counteract the reaction. The third medication gave me tinnitus, ringing in the ears. I reported this, but was told I was mistaken and it was the effects of the night before. With the second dose I experienced tinnitus and slight deafness. I was told that I was imagining this. 'After all what was worse, a UTI or the tinnitus?' I decided to accept the medication and flush it down the loo. I hoped to be discharged the next day and knew my GP would prescribe for me. I was very cross with myself for not checking on the second medication, and cross at not being treated for the infection earlier. I know my urinary problems very well and I would have liked to have been consulted earlier. I was discharged on the tenth day.

The first six weeks I had loss of sensation to pass urine, and resorted to a hot bath or lying flat on the floor for half an hour before going to the toilet. I was given a muscle relaxant. The consultant doesn't know why this happened. As I was in control it was decided to leave well alone for a few weeks. and then refer to a urologist if everything was still not normal. The seventh week I developed another urinary tract infection that responded to antibiotics. My GP visited weekly.

'Now two months post-op, I feel very positive, despite the setback with the bladder spasms and difficulty passing urine. I feel very well and am constantly told I look it. I really feel as if I am in control of myself. Sex has changed, but it has been enjoyable. Both of us were apprehensive the first couple of times. We are looking forward to the return of the very good sex life we had prior to my problems. I had no idea that I had adhesions or the damage they were doing until the operation. My wound has healed remarkably well and I am pleased with my post-op recovery.'

## JEAN

Jean, married for the second time, with three children by her first husband, had her total abdominal hysterectomy two years ago.

'I'd suffered with pain in my abdomen for several years. Various X-rays of small bowel and gall bladder, intravenous pylogram, barium meal, had revealed nothing wrong. The conclusion was that I had spastic colon or irritable bowel syndrome. I also had recurrent cystitis, which confused the issue even more. The bleeding at my monthly period was heavy, but I needed help for the pain.

'I was dismissed as being neurotic and left to my own devices. I tried wheat-free diets, herbal tablets, homeopathic pills, Bach flower remedies, even castor-oil poultice with a hot water bottle. It would have been possible to fry egg and bacon on my poor tummy, but no cure for THE PAIN. My elderly GP said it must be psychological and I played right into his hands, by crying. He couldn't see I was upset *because* of the pain, but he referred me, reluctantly, to the gynaecologist.

'Five months later, when the consultant touched my womb I almost leapt off the table, so great was the pain. He decided it was "time to remove this". I told him I didn't want any more children, and with a "Fine. We'll see you soon" he swept out and was seeing another patient before I was dressed. The nurse told me to "just go home and wait for a letter". I had no chance to ask the consultant anything. So many things raced around my head. Would it be a total or sub-total hysterectomy? Through the abdomen, or the vagina? Would I keep my ovaries and tubes? Someone had said in previous years that my right ovary was enlarged, but not why. I had been told absolutely nothing, there was a complete lack of information.

'I got in touch with HSG and was sent lots of helpful information and good advice. I bought two books and read up on the subject. I went to see my new GP, the other had retired, and asked was it being done to shut me up once and for all. He said no operation would be done for those reasons, and that some women were helped by the operation, some were not, it was my decision finally. I was glad that I was being taken seriously, but preferred the medical world to tell me I really needed it. I didn't want the responsibility!

'My biggest fear was the possibility of a blood clot. In bad moments, usually at night, I saw the operation going wrong with me ending up a cabbage, or worse still, my children orphans. I had pangs of guilt and at times considered not going through with it, because I owed it to my family to stay alive. In good moments I saw a new and pain-free life ahead of me. On the emotional side, I was sure that my husband and I would never be able to make love properly again and that he would find someone "normal". Fortunately, he reassured me and said that our love meant far more than just the physical side and I would be okay anyway. He had never wanted children of his own and had taken on my three children from my previous marriage, so this was not a problem. He knew something of hysterectomy, having seen a close member of his family go through it before we met. He was very understanding. The waiting made me anxious and it was ten months before the letter came telling me to go into hospital. The reality of it all struck me and I was scared.

'The hospital doctor who examined me mumbled and sniffed throughout and I could only pick up half of what he said. Mainly, if my ovaries were healthy I would not lose them. I told the young nurse that I was worried about a blood clot. She thought I'd be okay, but went off to ask the staff nurse who said I wasn't to worry about such things. Real assurance that! The consultant was new, the other had retired. Was I driving them all into retirement? He thought I was rather young to be having a hysterectomy and asked me if I was sure I wanted to go through with it? Well I had been preparing myself for the last ten months and did not intend to pack my case and go home at that stage! I said "I'm here now, so you may as well get on with it."

'Post-op I was in a lot of pain and had a urinary infection, so I felt low in spirits. I was told off for asking for the commode every half an hour, but ended up having a catheter for severe retention of urine. On the fifth day I was very weepy, but had no idea why I should feel that way. No one seemed to care and nobody reassured me that all these feelings were a normal follow-up. As a whole my experience in hospital was very bad so I was glad when ten days post-op I was able to go home.

'Surprisingly, I found myself in tears on arrival back home, though I don't know why. I felt scared being away from immediate medical help and suddenly everything seemed so strange. I felt totally detached from the normal world. My post-op appointment was in seven weeks time with nobody to see me before. As it happened my GP visited a couple of days later as the urinary infection returned. At the post-op check, I was told that the laboratory test on my womb was okay, so I still do not know what caused the pain. None of my feelings or worries were treated seriously and I was expected to go along with everything, ask no questions and 'be a good girl'. If only the doctors and nurses had taken time out, just five minutes each time, to ask how I *really* felt.

'Two years on, I get aches associated with a "knot of stitch" on my right side, but the consultants are reluctant to do anything. I do not regret having the hysterectomy done. It is lovely not to have monthly problems or any pain in between. Fears about making love were unfounded. My one regret is that thousands of women are still treated as I was, just a name on a list and not a woman with feelings.'

## ALICE

Alice, married with three children, had a total abdominal hysterectomy a year ago, at 30. Alice came to England from West Africa, with her husband, five years ago. Her two elder children remained in Africa with her parents. Alice was sterilized for health reasons after her third child was born, four years ago.

'After this it was a bad time for me. I sent my daughter home to Africa, she was a year old. I had much bleeding and much pain and had different treatments from the doctors. Nothing was of help and after eighteen months I went into hospital for a hysterectomy. My husband also felt this was the best thing and was very kind. I recovered very quick in hospital, but things were different when I came home. I felt most tired and was very weak and ill. I thought of the children I would not have. All my children are girls and I had wanted sons as well and now it was too late. It was very final and I was saddened to tears. I felt no longer a woman, useless, and a hindrance to my husband, who was still a young man. I was a shell, withered and dried inside.

'My husband was still kind, but didn't understand how I felt. I told him I was finished, he would have to take another wife and he was angry. I went to my own room and no longer shared bed or food with him. It is the way of my people, but my husband did not accept this. He said our culture may say finish, no womb, but he feel that individuals do it differently. I had no feel for sex as there would be no more children. He knew there was not another man. I cried many days, but grew strong in mind. I knew what was right to do and that when I had gone my husband would find another woman to mother his sons.

'The hysterectomy has taken the pain and I am strong. I have turned my face from the life that was and will return to Africa and my family there.'

## ANNETTE

Annette, married, but childless, had a total abdominal hysterectomy when 29. Annette is registered disabled and has problems with mobility.

'It was revealed at a genetic counselling session that my

grandparents were first cousins and that, due to this, my mother, their only child, was blind. My sister and myself were left with a progressive cerebral lesion of which there was little evidence, but the deterioration once started would be fairly rapid. There was a one in two chance of us having a handicapped child. I was then 17, pregnant, and had just had German measles, so decided to have a termination. Later on I could think more positively about the future and whether I wanted to bring another handicapped child into the world.

'At 24 I married the man of my dreams. We had decided that we wouldn't have children and my husband had a vasectomy. Eighteen months later it was discovered that I'd had an accidental overdose of radioactive iodine when treated for a severe thyroid condition at 21. The side effect was the destruction of the hormone system. I felt bitter about this, as I had extremely heavy, painful periods. I used to flood and needed to change every hour, at night I used disposable nappies. I had a fourteen-day cycle with just four days when I felt well. The rest were spent in pain, feeling sick and depressed with frequent bouts of tiredness. So I wasn't very keen on going out and sex was just a four-letter word. My GP had never been interested in the bleeding, but he referred me to a consultant when I asked. During those four years, I had two D and Cs and two lots of hormone tablets. The two years before my operation were really bad. I could hardly bear to be touched, my stomach and breasts used to ache so much, even the water from the shower was uncomfortable. We were lucky if we made love twice a month.

'Hysterectomy was in the news. I'd read a magazine article about it and heard a famous singer and television personality talk about her hysterectomy. I looked it up at the Department of Health and Social Security (DHSS) library and decided to ask for the op at my next hospital appointment. I went determined to get my own way and took a friend for moral support. The doctor also had the same idea, but was not sure how I would take it. We laugh about it now as I waited until she was doing the obligatory internal, before asking quite calmly "Please. Can I just have a hysterectomy?" I got dressed and we discussed it over coffee! Was this the NHS? All my questions about the operation, time in hospital, the scar etc. were answered there and then. I would go on the waiting list and if in three months time I still wanted to go ahead, I was to write and let her know. So I was looking at four months at the most. For once I was being treated like a woman that knew her own mind and not like a glorified member of a cattle market. I went home feeling really great. After all that time I had been taken seriously.

'Although I didn't regard it as major surgery, my husband did. He felt it was a risk worth taking if it made me better. I'd been promised a bikini cut if I lost weight, so I swam a lot, lost two stone in weight and got super fit. I had difficulty walking by this time and periodically had to use a wheelchair. I was really worried about walking after the operation and talked to my GP about this. He was the most unsympathetic, pig ignorant man that I have ever met. He asked me if it really mattered!! He said: "Go home, don't think about it, after all you'll be asleep when they do it."

'I was admitted to hospital, prepared and sent to theatre. When I came round in the ward, no operation had been done, as the lift to theatre had broken down! I just cried and cried. I was sent home and re-admitted a week later. Going into hospital was really easy for me and I told a nurse that this was no worse than having my appendix out! That afternoon I had a visit from the hospital social worker who drew a little diagram for me to make sure I knew what was going on. When I went to theatre I was terrified the lift would break down again. It didn't, but the next thing I knew it was two days later. I had haemorrhaged on returning to the ward after the op and they had kept me sedated to stop the bleeding. Getting out of bed the first time was the worst part. I thought I might burst my one, four-inch stitch! The scar looks just like a stretch mark now. I recovered well and went home in seven days. Apart from a little infection at the vault of the vagina, which took three weeks to clear, I had no problems. The bleeding stopped in three weeks and I was told I could try a gentle swim a week later. At the post-op check I was warned that although my ovaries had been left I might need HRT in ten years' time.

'After losing all that weight I discovered a figure that men obviously found attractive. I became more confident, but my husband had difficulty in adjusting. He was afraid of hurting me and wouldn't touch me after the hysterectomy. I tried, I really did, but in the end I went out and experimented with a particular man. I'm not proud of it but I did enjoy sex with him. Forbidden fruit maybe, but I felt wanted for a few months until my husband got over his fear. My husband never found out and sex is far more enjoyable now than it has ever been. We have been married ten years, have a very good relationship and I still love him.

'I seemed to sail through, happy it was all over and at last I could get on with living my life. I did not feel any resentment, but eight months later, my best friend had just had a baby and my mother took great delight in telling me my sister was having another. My mother had never once asked how I felt about not having any children. It suddenly struck me just what I had been through and I could not tell a soul just how hurt I felt. In a way I suppose I felt sorry for myself, or maybe it was just a grieving process, a natural mourning for the children I could never have. I rang HSG. Someone listened to me and just said "Hey, yes, it is alright for you to feel like this." I was so upset, I only heard the voice, but it made sense.

'Three years later I really am over it. I don't hurt inside any more and often visit my friends with kids and do things with them. My walking has improved, I use crutches and don't need a wheelchair any more. I have lost some more weight and still swim, fitting into the smallest of bikinis. I now work full time, but even more important, I do little things for me. I have started HRT and feel GREAT.'

## JANE

Jane, married with two grown-up children, had a total abdominal hysterectomy two years ago.

'I never thought I'd need a hysterectomy. I had reached the age of 50 without having any gynaecological problems. After a long and heavy bleed a D and C diagnosed hyperplasia (overgrowth of the lining of the womb) but I was convinced that the progesterone tablets would do the trick, and they did. I was surprised when friends asked why I was bothering with "all that" and why didn't I have a hysterectomy? It seemed the easier option to have a little bottle of pills to take if the bleeding got out of hand. Easier than waiting for an appointment with the gynaecologist each time, but the gynaecologist explained that the second course was all I could have. Had I thought of having a hysterectomy? The onus was on me. He would understand if I was fed up, and would do the operation if I asked for it.

'I went back to work wondering How can I decide this? My husband had been very worried by my suddenly malfunctioning gynaecology, and thought asking for a hysterectomy difficult for me to do. The next day I went to the coast for a day on my own and walked and thought about it. The surgeon was moving hospitals, I wanted him to do it before he went, and my daughter was getting married in eight months' time. If I was going to have the operation, I needed to have it quickly. The surgeon had other ways of filling his time and wouldn't have offered surgery had it not been a good idea. So that was it!

'My husband was sympathetic and thought that the operation was the best idea, but understood that it was a decision I hadn't wanted to make. I was unable to compose the letter asking for it, so we did it together.

'The operation date was three weeks later. The surgeon went out of his way to assure me that it was the best thing and the actual surgery was splendid and painless. The hospital was surprised at my rapid recovery and described it as remarkable. I had a high on the fourth day post-op, sort of born again. It was sooner than I had expected.

'Five weeks later I didn't feel so good. I remember vividly the "black cloak descending" feeling. It was a shock. The physical healing was impressive and I hadn't reckoned with having depression at all. The hospital information sheet said that six weeks after surgery you should be back to normal. When everything had gone so well, it sounded like whingeing to say depression was really bothersome. The fact was noted, but given cursory attention, beyond being prescribed HRT for the low moods and flushes which had also begun. Time passed and I looked well. It was difficult to mention depression.

'I had my daughter's wedding to arrange and was feeling desperate about the bridesmaids' dresses. While shopping, I suddenly felt so exhausted I could have laid down between all the milling shoppers, with no comfort at all, and considered it bliss. Three months after the hysterectomy, I increasingly had a lack of energy and enthusiasm and began to feel quite antisocial at times. Feelings of exhaustion could hit out of the blue and I began to find it all rather upsetting. I felt cheated and under pressure to put on a good face. Relatives and friends were a source of annoyance by their cheerful insistence that I looked "so well since having that op". Dragging up a positive response was difficult. When I felt upset the scar was slightly uncomfortable too.

'My husband, aware that I wasn't as bright as I looked, arranged things that I normally enjoyed doing, but realized it didn't help. Nor did the flowers, the perfume, the hair do's . . . all the things you're patted on the head and told to do. I was looking well and according to friends, ten years younger. I hinted that I'd had some downers, but I felt they were dismissive, so I was unable to say more. I became skilful at acting when times were bad.

'The operation experience affected my whole body image to some degree. There was nothing to see, but in a vague way I no longer felt quite comfortable with myself. Previously positive about buying clothes, I was often undecided and wondered if something I had bought was

29

really me. The new modern hairstyle made me look more like my mother and aunts, and I wasn't entirely happy on that score. Sexually I was a reluctant participant. It was the thought of it more than anything else. I read that gynaecologists used to try and leave the cervix because women missed it. I think that's true as I thought of myself as sexually different.

'The depth of the depression surprised me. I was unable to make any positive gesture which might have been helpful. This was odd, because on other levels I was still able to function efficiently. It was a well-kept secret and in that way was quite isolating. Sometimes super cheerful and energetic, sometimes extremely lethargic and depressed, I needed help to deal with this roller-coaster style of life. My doctor would save my life in a physical emergency, but I wouldn't get a sympathetic hearing, if I said I was fed up. Especially as this lady had said I'd feel born anew after hysterectomy.

'I read about psychotherapy and counselling in a newspaper. The articles were informative and reassuring, so I pursued the idea. I felt counselling was rather un-British and didn't want to talk to anyone about it and so it was some time before I found a service. Then I had doubts about keeping the appointment and felt quite threatened. I kept in mind that therapists were non-judgemental and try to offer a secure and trusting relationship. When the time came I did feel just bad enough to go. It was a year after my hysterectomy.

'I was very uptight that first time, but the counsellor's relaxed, attentive listening seemed to be the height of generosity. "I hear what you say and it matters." Many of us have never been truly listened to in our lives. The experience is a bit like drowning. Life's events are inclined to flash by and one thing you talk about can revive others. We have no control over the rate or time that bad experiences hit us and I was able to view a whole series of events. Both my children marrying and leaving home during the same time as four friends dying, a relative, feeling completely overcome by health worries, seeking support from me, my husband's cardiac problems, my own heavy workload, the hysterectomy. Also memories of my mother, many years ago, insisting it was selfish to be depressed. If one thought of others there wouldn't be time for depression! I told of the great feelings of sadness since the hysterectomy. The counsellor said that it was all right and why didn't I cry about it? I was surprised, it was a relief to hear, but I've never actually been able to cry. My mother felt as strongly about crying as she did about depression and father claimed such people had their bladder too near their eyes!

'The sexual experience is now good, but brings feelings of sadness to the fore. To begin with I did think in terms of getting back to normal and I applied this to everything, but you change after any major experience and this can be all right. To act as though it hasn't happened isn't a positive thing to do. My experience has bothered me, especially the contrast of outward show and inward feelings. Is it coincidence that such feelings should occur following hysterectomy? Would the same have happened after other surgery? What about the monumental implications of the equivalent operation on a man? How would it affect his personality and feelings of sexuality? Everyone would expect big problems to be worked through and a great deal of adjusting to take place! This should be considered when ladies undergo hysterectomy. A dilemma! Might the surgeon replace physical pain with psychological pain? It seems terrible to suggest they do and logically shouldn't happen. The removal of a troublesome organ, no longer required should have nothing but beneficial results. (Of course, the event is a cause for celebration for some.) There seems to be no reason to feel depleted sexually, or as a person, or that it's an ageing experience, or you have a figure that isn't yours, or all sorts of odd things that ladies will admit to if pressed on the matter. It is totally unhelpful to give this aspect scant recognition, or worse still, no recognition at all, or to blame the women. To say how it *could* be doesn't mean that it *will* be so. It should be acknowledged that some ladies feel incredible loss and grief about losing their uterus; that it is all right to feel that way. Why not reassure that in time, ladies come to terms with it and the pain fades?

'Was hysterectomy worth it for me? The thought persists that at my age the bleeding might have stopped any time of it's own accord. Even now I feel some pressure to say "It's all marvellous". To be honest, I don't feel joyous about the hysterectomy and don't see myself ever feeling that. But then I guess it's all right not to.

'Those quiet and wise Chinese have a very old saying: "This too will pass." Here is a not-so-quiet, or wise, English lady who agrees. And adds – GOOD!'

# 3.
# FIBROIDS

Heavy, painful bleeding may be the first sign of fibroids, a term that is more familiar to women than the medical names, myoma or fibromyoma. They are non-cancerous lumps of the womb and usually grow quite slowly over a period of years. Most develop no further than the walls of the womb, but some carry on growing to protrude into the womb or the pelvic cavity. A few develop a stalk, or may grow in the broad ligament or cervix. Each type has a different name and several can and often do grow at the same time, producing a large, heavy mass. The weight of this or a large fibroid, leaning on the bladder, bowel, womb or other pelvic organs, can produce pressure symptoms that need treatment. Fibroids do not always give problems and many women have them without knowing. They are very common, 5 per cent of all women have them, and they are the reason for a large number of hysterectomies. Size is usually measured in terms of a pregnant uterus (womb) and for those over 12 weeks an abdominal hysterectomy is usually done. One of the six women in this chapter had a vaginal hysterectomy as her fibroid was fairly small.

Three of the women are single and childless, three are married with children and the age range is from 35 to 52.

## IONA

Iona, married with one daughter, had a total abdominal hysterectomy at 43, four years ago.

'My periods had always been irregular, slight and painless, but suddenly they became regular, heavy and painful. For six months my GP tried various treatments and then referred me to a gynaecologist. A D and C made things worse, and a hysterectomy was suggested. I felt unsure about this; removal of my womb seemed a bit drastic, but it was true that I didn't want any more children. I could not feel that the removal of a useless organ would make me feel less feminine. A talk with my lady GP was reassuring, although I realized afterwards that she had told me very little that was factual. One remark she made was incredible and made me laugh even then. "Do not worry about sex afterwards, my dear, your husband will notice no difference"!

'So I was admitted to hospital for a hysterectomy. The surgeon and anaesthetist explained things briefly, but I was perfectly calm about it all simply because I understood so little. I had no knowledge of major operations at all. I had told my husband and daughter as much as I knew, and we had tried to prepare adequately at home, but none of us were at all worried.

'When I came to after the operation, I realized that the pain in my back had gone. I had grown so used to it I scarcely noticed it – but I noticed its disappearance. I made steady progress and my wound healed well and I remember the kind nurses, cheerful patients, exhausting visitors, and agonizing wind pains on walking. The surgeon explained that a large fibroid on the outside of my womb had pressed on my spine, causing the backache. There wasn't any malignancy. I cheerfully went home after ten days.

'I was quite unprepared for the pain, tiredness, inadequacy and bad nights which hit me at home. I survived and gradually began to feel better. I was helped by contact with a voluntary group, HSG. I was very fortunate in having a helpful husband, who coped well and gave me breakfast in bed every day for three months. I had a remarkably straightforward operation and a smooth recovery.

'After the six-week check-up, one is supposed to return to work and sex. I found contemplating sex very difficult, as I could not bear the thought of hurting or even touching.

my tummy. Fortunately my husband was very patient and I soon found our sex life much more enjoyable. The GP's prediction was true – my husband notices no difference!! I know that my vagina must be shorter, it really does feel different to me, but I'm used to it now and do not mind. The feeling that my tummy was sensitive and vulnerable, lasted for about two years.

'In about three months I was perfectly restored and was walking, driving, and working. I didn't have my ovaries removed and haven't had any aftereffects. My scar has now faded and all I feel is the continuing relief of no periods and no contraception.

'We knew so little. I was unable to warn my daughter about the drips and tubes immediately post-op. She was horrified at the sight of it all. The effect was rather detrimental and her behaviour became wild and deceitful. She did badly at O-level and went on to fail dismally at A-level. A year after my operation, she told of her fear, unexpressed at the time, that I was dying. I do wonder, if I had known more and prepared her better for my operation, whether things might have been better, steadier for her. Also, a close friend watched my easy recovery and she, too, went ahead and had a hysterectomy. In her case there were problems from which she never recovered.

I advise anyone facing a major operation to have a much more responsible and knowledgeable attitude than I had. More counselling should be available, so that the whole family can be prepared for drips, tubes, tears and all the rest of it. Then perhaps everyone in the family would feel the benefit as much as I did.'

## MARTHA

Martha, single and childless, had a total abdominal hysterectomy with removal of both ovaries at 42, nearly two years ago. Martha has received treatment for epilepsy since the age of 11. She maintained a full-time job while living at home looking after her elderly frail parents. A few months after her menstrual symptoms, due to fibroids, had worsened and Martha was on long-term sick leave, her mother died.

'My menstrual problems of flooding with clots and bleeding without an hour's break, had gradually worsened. I became anaemic and had to sit with my feet up for six months. The recent and unexpected loss of my mother meant that besides my own physical problems, I was thrown into a new, difficult, strange and tragic situation. We had been a very close-knit family, but women's troubles and problems had never ever been discussed. It was especially difficult and distressing for Father, as I am the daughter many years his junior, and not his wife – very embarrassing on both sides. I had to be the "strong" partner, which was very difficult.

'When a hysterectomy was suggested I had a vague idea of what it meant, but the thought didn't bother me. Many women feel that they lose their womanhood after the operation, but I saw it as a change of state in a woman's life. I had mixed feelings about a major operation and was in a terrible state going to theatre – nerves, tears, worry and fright. I had a slight epileptic attack on coming round after this, but all they had done was a D and C!! So I was pleased and relieved, as was my father, when four months later the hysterectomy was going to take place. We both hoped that most of my troubles would be over and I couldn't get there quickly enough. I was upset at the thought of losing my ovaries and felt that I was "conned" into this part. The hospital doctor was praised for managing to persuade me to agree, but I hadn't much choice or say in the matter.

'I worried, not about the anaesthetic but about gallstones, and the fear of thrombosis was great. My mother's recent death had been due to thrombosis. I did in fact come out of hospital with white pressure stockings on my legs. Losing my ovaries also worried me with regard to breast cancer and osteoporosis.

'Post-op I was thrilled it was all over. I hadn't realized how little I knew until this op; it was like an adventure into the unknown. All of us in the ward were going through it together, and were able to help each other. For forty-eight hours after the operation I had hallucinations, especially at night, which was frightening. The other frightening situation was to be discharged after eight days with no chance of convalescence. One is thrown into a home environment with literally nothing, not even a district nurse. No real advice was given about how to cope on leaving hospital at all. I returned home unable to do anything and it was atrocious that my recently bereaved, elderly father was expected to do it all. In my father's generation, it was wrong to ask for help of any kind, no mention was ever to be made of one's troubles. One literally had to "grin and bear it". No true feelings were ever to be shown and a person had to push themselves. My father was worried that he was going to lose me in the same way that he had so recently lost his wife. As I came out of hospital, he contracted a bronchial virus which lasted for eight weeks. I was so worried that I was going to lose him. It was a very difficult and frustrating time. What shocked us both is that people we had expected to rally round, didn't. The surprise was that friends appeared from the most unexpected quarters and the experience has brought us closer together.

'If *only* the HRT would work! I am now on my fifth type of HRT. I would be so pleased if I could feel well and not act like "a little old lady of 90". The drugs for epilepsy are strong and it is difficult for the HRT to break through. It is hard to obtain the right balance and strength of drugs. It appears to be very much trial and error, especially as they cause so many different and frustrating side effects. What is so frightening is to be told that if you do not have HRT you will get osteoporosis and if you do have HRT you will have gallstones, thrombosis or breast cancer. One feels condemned before you start! People keep saying "You will feel a new woman, ten to twenty years younger" or "You'll look so well!" Well I'm still waiting and hoping that I will not have to wait much longer before I see and feel like the "new me"! I still do not understand why the ovaries had to be removed. I did not appreciate the full extent of the operation, especially regarding losing the ovaries, HRT and epilepsy.

'The operation was of some benefit: no periods, no pain and no pre-menstrual tension. It is a luxury not to have to carry around a big shopping bag filled up with three complete changes of clothes, washing kit, sanitary towels, etcetera. It is sheer bliss not to have to answer questions on why I have to carry such a big heavy bag all the time! The hysterectomy just finalized everything regarding children, being unmarried and the age I was. It has made no difference at all to my sex life, which is of little importance. I am pleased that it was done, and would go through it again.'

## LOUISE

Louise, single, and childless, had a total abdominal hysterectomy at 33, four years ago. Louise was in a stable relationship at the time, working and running her own flat. Her immediate family live many miles away. Louise is blind.

'Some years ago after a D and C and laparotomy, I was told I had fibroids and could go back if they caused any problems. Five years later, I was considering sterilization as I didn't want children. The doctor suggested hysterectomy since the fibroids, now much larger, were causing pain and heavy bleeding. I knew about the operation and welcomed it to relieve the symptoms. I am disabled and I felt that my womb, described by doctors as bulky and misshapen, was causing me further handicap. I definitely did not want children, so felt that I could live better without it.

'The hospital doctor was particularly careful to make sure that I wanted the hysterectomy, but was bad at explaining the operation and after care. After the hysterectomy, I lay in hospital wondering where this thing, my womb, had gone. Was it lying in a bin somewhere? What would happen to it?

'My boyfriend finds hospitals quite frightening, but he

came to see me. He never asked how I was, as he already knew – he had sympathetic pains. The nurses were very caring and sensitive, but the doctors less so. The woman registrar had been approachable in Out Patients, but her ward visits were brief and provided little opportunity for asking questions. The consultant never came. The house officer had difficulty in communicating with me, and I felt my blindness greatly embarrassed him. He would arrive and pull the curtains around the bed, lift back the bed clothes and begin to examine me without saying a word. His brisk manner and failure to explain his actions frightened and humiliated me. All this left me feeling that I had been mutilated and that I had betrayed a part of my body by allowing it to be removed.

'I was discharged home after seven days with a leaflet about immediate symptoms. Although very tired I made a good recovery physically, but the experience of being dependent in an unfamiliar environment left emotional and mental scars. I went for convalescence to stay with older friends, but I was unable to talk things through with them. People kept saying that I was very young to have the operation. The strong religious view was that I was single and shouldn't have had a hysterectomy. I felt guilty I'd had the operation and criticized for allowing it. I came home to be on my own. I was very tearful.

'At the six-week post-operation check, there were different doctors. I had a pain in my side and was told it was only bruising. I needed to talk to someone, and went to see the ward sister, but it was very busy, so I didn't bother. I had been warned that although I would be well by six weeks, it would be six months before I was full of energy. I went back to work at seven weeks, but was extremely tired. I had never been so tired and the pain in my side continued. I began to realize that the choice of not having children was different to not being able to have children. My main problem seemed to be a changed body image with a possible loss of sexuality. My mother, many miles away, felt it was all a lot of nonsense.

'Four months post-op my doctor was treating me for

depression and I was admitted to hospital. In fact, I was so tired, they just observed me and looked after me while I rested for two weeks. While in hospital I had a very heavy vaginal discharge and passed clots of blood. I was told it was debris from the operation and the pain in my side went. The physiotherapist at this hospital was very helpful and very good. I felt much better on discharge, but it took me about a year to work through the emotional and mental problems.

'Three things helped me overcome them. Firstly, my *sexual* confidence was restored with help from my boyfriend. He kept his distance until I was ready and was very careful not to hurt me. Sex is different. You have to forget what it was like before and find out about how it is now. Some things are much more pleasurable. Secondly, *talking things through* and getting information was invaluable. The HSG gave information and a sympathetic listener. I had lost part of my body and was grieving for my womb. I would grieve for any bit of me that was removed. Thirdly, I symbolically "*buried*" my womb in the coffin at my father's funeral! Bizarre, I know, but it helped heal all the hurts. Finally I was able to lay it to rest.

'Now I have no regrets. I am healthier, my skin is better, I'm not anaemic and my backache is gone.'

## ROBBIE

Robbie, single and childless, had a total abdominal hysterectomy at 40, two years ago. Robbie, a trained health professional, was without a partner at the time of her operation. Her widowed father lives a distance away. Robbie was told three years before that she had fibroids, that her womb was the size of a 14-week pregnancy and that she needed a hysterectomy.

'My GP had said "it's a useless uterus!" and that if I'd been ten years younger they would have saved the uterus, and if I'd been ten years older they'd certainly not bother to do so! He would normally refer for a hysterectomy, but because of my age, 37, and my reluctance to have the operation, he would refer me to a women's hospital.

'I walked home barely able to hold back the tears and then I cried solidly for three hours. I no sooner stopped than I started again. I felt it was so unfair to happen at my age, before I'd ever had children. Now it seemed I'd never have the chance to. I felt my life was over and that no one would ever want me again. I felt a freak. Other women of 37 don't suffer this. I felt it was the worst day of my life.

'I bought a textbook on gynaecology, so I would understand what the consultant said to his students in technical terms. I had a strong need to see what fibroids looked like and went to an anatomical museum. I found it reassuring in a strange way. I could see that it would be impossible to become pregnant – there would be no room left inside for a foetus. I was also reassured to see that fibroids looked much less horrible than I had imagined them. This led to my regarding them as something that was a growing part of me, rather than the distasteful invasion of my womb that I had imagined.

'The emotional pain of the coming loss was far harder to deal with. The pain was nearly too much to bear, I felt grief-stricken and too choked to eat. My youth, my options, my physiological destiny in life, my womanhood – suddenly all were dead. I felt flung overnight from a young person to being a late middle-aged one, an utter failure. Any reminders, such as babies crying or hearing that a 47-year-old woman had got pregnant accidentally, while I couldn't do it on purpose, sent me into floods of tears again. Everyone seemed to have young children or were pregnant. I was desperately envious of them all.

'It turned me right off men and I began to hate them. I was sure I would never ever want sex again after what was happening to my body. What was the point of sex or relationships now, when they could no longer lead to marriage and children? I cut this aspect entirely out of my life for five years.

'I went home for the weekend to tell my father. He

remarked that my mother had had the same trouble, but a myomectomy had been possible and she'd gone on to conceive afterwards. He let me read a series of letters that she had written to him at a time when she was trying to conceive and was faced with the fact that she might have to have a hysterectomy. I found them moving and wished my mother was there to talk to. My father was very upset, it meant no grandchildren. He later confided in his sister, who said that she was not telling anyone, as if it was a shameful secret. To me she said: "You're a sensible, strong girl, you'll get over it all right, we all have to face these things." That was nearly as useless a response as my doctor's. He had reminded me I was nearly 40 and that the menopause wasn't far off. Was that supposed to make me feel better?

'The consultant arranged an ultra-sound scan and I saw one very large fibroid and several small ones. As I preferred to delay the operation the consultant saw me at six-monthly intervals for the next three years. By which time I'd put on four inches around the waist, a stone in weight and had bladder problems. The uterus was now the size of a 20-week pregnancy. There was a small, but increasing risk of malignant change and I reluctantly agreed to the hysterectomy being performed. It almost broke my heart. There was no question of myomectomy and I would have to have a vertical incision.

'I can't count how many people told me I'd feel "a new woman" after the op and would wish I'd had it done years ago. A good few also threw the old cliché at me that "it wouldn't affect your femininity or your sexual enjoyment". That was the last thing I cared about at the time. I soon realized it was better to only confide in the trusted few who could understand. Such people, with letters and offers of help, did much to keep me going.

'I was secretly in tears several times during the admission day and then the pre-med injection dried them up. So I cried dry, soundless, wrenching tears listening to the sound of children in a school playground at the back of the hospital building. I wrote in my diary: "I should be on cloud nine, from the injection, but I'm not. I just have a headache and a heartache as I say goodbye to my body, goodbye youth forever.'

'Post-operatively I was looked after very well by an excellent team of doctors and nurses. Pain was well controlled by injections and pills. I was in hospital for two weeks and never once felt any emotional reaction to the loss of my uterus. I still had my ovaries, but I didn't seem to care any more about the hysterectomy. It hit me about a month later, when I fell into a terrible depression and cried day after day for several weeks.

'It is eighteen months since the operation and it has been a difficult time. So traumatic in fact that I would never have had the operation done, ever, if I had realized the emotional repercussions. Hysterectomy has brought me no benefit whatsoever. I have a hard, pink, keloid scar almost half an inch wide extending down my abdomen and this distresses me a great deal. My bladder has never returned to the pre-frequency stage. I still suffer with the physical symptoms of pre-menstrual tension and at times severe cramps where my uterus used to be. I miss my periods, because I'm not like other young women. When I finally resumed sex recently, it was at first downright impossible and then extremely painful. Most important of all is how hysterectomy (contrary to what they all tell you) has affected the way in which I see myself. Post-operation, I was left feeling like a 60-year-old, looking only to the end of her life. It is just in the past few weeks that I have even started to feel anywhere like my present age of 41. That has come about through the kindness and understanding of a man who cares about me as a person and who can share with me the tragedy of this operation.'

## SHEILA

Sheila, married with two grown-up children, had a total abdominal hysterectomy, with both ovaries removed, at 52, six years ago. Sheila's problems began with flooding and blood clots two years prior to surgery.

'I had been on different types of iron tablets and had suffered from anaemia over the last few years. My GP sent me to a gynaecologist and I had a D and C, which showed small fibroids. I was counselled by the consultant about having a hysterectomy. I was more than happy to have done with the constant tiredness, flooding and general expense of pads. I wanted it done as soon as possible to get rid of the misery of going out to dinner, working, driving, and finding myself with a bloodstained skirt.

'As a nurse, I knew what the operation meant and I had help from my nurse daughter, the consultant and my GP. A nurse colleague, who'd just had a hysterectomy, was so well and feeling so much better that she encouraged me, as did my boss who'd also had a hysterectomy for fibroids that year. The thought of the operation did not worry me.

'The family felt the sooner it was done, the better. They were fed up with a tired, weepy woman about the house, but my operation was postponed. There was a work-to-rule and I had a phone call saying no bed! I rang the consultant and a bed was found. On admission I had to wait and see if there was a bed; there was. This was very upsetting and all the fears I didn't have until then, appeared. I had blood tests after lunch, but the anaesthetist came at 8 p.m. and the house physician at 11 p.m. I've mentioned these points as I'm sure that had I been a lay person, I would have been in a worse state than I was. Reassurance and advice at 11 p.m. was a bit late as a pre-op exercise, to say the least. We had to ask advice from the doctors, especially regarding travel and sex. My husband had had an arteriogram the day before, following a severe heart attack six months previously. There was surprise from fellow patients that we requested to see the houseman together.

'Post-op I was not prepared to find myself with a drip – as I had needed blood – or a drainage tube. The night sister was aware of pain relief and gave me pain killers before my pain threshold reached its peak and before I was washed. She was gentle and very kind. Other post-op patients on other nights did not get this consideration. I was lucky, it was her last night on duty before she went on holiday.

'The nursing auxiliary read my chart and told me I'd had my ovaries removed! I asked about hormone replacement therapy and the Greek registrar raised his eyebrows. He said that having ovaries removed at my age was okay as I didn't want to have more children, did I? He didn't understand. I had a wound infection and remained in hospital for fourteen days. My consultant said that he had removed my ovaries as there was such a mess inside, it would save him having to operate again in a few years. He was helpful and advised HRT.

'On return home my GP visited me the next day and I commenced HRT tablets, which I took for three years before coming off them. I became so miserable and tetchy that my GP put me on them again. I took them for another two years and then came off them gradually, and this is by far the best way. I have been off HRT for nearly two years and feel fine.

'At present I have a good sex life. I am told that I look about 50 years and not nearly 60 years. My skin is smooth with hardly any wrinkles. I feel great!'

## CAROL

Carol, married with two children, had a total vaginal hysterectomy two years ago, at 35.

'After the birth of my second baby, four years ago, I began to get heavy, irregular bleeding with backache. I also had difficulties sorting out contraception. My husband and I felt sterilization was a good idea as our family was now complete, and I went to see a specialist. After the examination, the specialist said I had a small fibroid, about the size of a walnut, and also a slight prolapse of the womb. He felt that the fibroid was probably causing the bleeding difficulties. He suggested that I go home and discuss the possibility of a hysterectomy with my husband rather than have a sterilization. He told me where to get information on hysterectomy and suggested I talked to his nurse counsellor.

'The next visit, my husband came with me and the specialist answered all our questions and explained all we wanted to know. He was very helpful, as was my GP. Hysterectomy was known to me as my mother had had one for a prolapse and I remember it made a great improvement for her.

'I had the op four months later and was well looked after in a ward with several other ladies having hysterectomies. I found that I made a quicker recovery than the women who'd had abdominal cuts. I had a catheter direct into the bladder above my pubic bone and also vaginal packing/dressing. These were a bit unexpected, but were removed after two days with no trouble at all. I continued to make a good recovery. They had taken my womb, cervix, small fibroid and also performed a vaginal repair. I was discharged home after six days with instructions on lifting and exercises from the hospital physiotherapist for the next three months. My backache was gone.

'We paid a home help to come in twice a week for twelve weeks and my sister came every day for a while to help with the children. My husband was very supportive, as was my mother.

'I had a little pot belly for a while, but when that went I was pleased not to have a visible scar on my tummy. The only worry I did have was that as I'd had blood I might get AIDS. My GP spent a long time explaining the process of collecting blood, the tests that are made and how the blood is treated. He explained in detail, and how imported blood in the past had caused problems, but was no longer used. Of course I've been so well since the op, I feel a bit of a fool to have worried about it.

'I think I did so well because I had the op before any of my symptoms became really troublesome and dragged me down. I felt really well at four months and haven't looked back since. I have no regrets as some women have. I haven't felt depressed, anxious or concerned about my sex life, which has improved since the op.'

# 4.
# ENDOMETRIOSIS AND ADENOMYOSIS

The endometrium is the lining of the womb and in response to the ovarian hormones, it builds up each month to receive a fertilized egg. If the egg is not fertilized, it passes out of the body and the lining of the womb sheds in a monthly bleed. *Endometriosis* is when the lining of the womb is present in other sites of the body, usually the bladder, bowel, vagina and pelvic areas. It responds in the same way to the ovarian hormones, causing discomfort, heavy, painful periods, painful intercourse and various other symptoms. Chocolate cysts may form on the ovaries, while fibroids, adhesions and inflammation also seem common occurrences. The amount of endometriosis and associated symptoms varies from woman to woman. This chapter looks at three women with endometriosis and three with *adenomyosis*. This is the occurrence of endometriosis in the muscle of the womb, which may be the only site of endometriosis. Several of the women had a variety of symptoms. Five are married with children and one is childless; age range 31 to 42.

## BRENDA

Brenda, married with four children, had an abdominal hysterectomy at 39, five months ago. Problems began seven years ago, after the birth of her fourth child, her only daughter. For four years she ignored her symptoms, putting the family first. Her daughter needed a lot of attention, encephalitis at 10 months had left her with minor epileptic (petit mal) fits. Her husband was unemployed through illness and the elder boys were unsettled and demanding.

'I started to go down hill. Each period I dreaded, each month I hated and, feeling ill, I couldn't cope any longer. My GP referred me to the consultant. After a laparoscopy diagnosed endometriosis, I asked for a hysterectomy, but was told I wasn't bad enough and they only did it when really necessary. I had a course of Danazol capsules to stop my periods. I felt great, but began having side effects, bad headaches and feeling sick. I came off them and was back to square one. I persevered another three years like that. I had post-natal depression after my third baby and I was still, after all this time, suffering from depression. I nursed my sister who had cancer, until she died. We were very close. Then we had a house fire and lost everything and that knocked me for six. My doctor said I was heading for a nervous breakdown. I put a lot of this down to my illness, not just physically, but mentally too. I felt sorry for myself, for my husband, too. I was terrible to him, arguing all the time, the least little thing set me off. He was very supportive, and kept asking what could he do; he wasn't a woman, he didn't understand. What a life! It was no life, just surviving! Looking back there's strength coming from somewhere to keep us together as a family.

'My doctor put me on hormone tablets and within six months I had put on three stone in weight! I asked to see the consultant again and went the next month. Within two minutes of him examining me he asked me to go in for a hysterectomy. I couldn't believe what he said. The relief that word was to me. Nine weeks later I had my operation.

'I cannot tell you the *relief* I felt on the day of the operation. I was so happy. Two days later I was up and walking around. I felt fantastic, no backache, no nothing. I felt re-born, alive. My husband had a shock when he saw me. He expected me to look ill, but my colour had come back in my face. I felt great. To get rid of backache and stomach pain after seven years was unbelievable. LIFE AT LAST!

'The second week at home, I felt depressed and very low. I am a person who goes here, there and everywhere, shopping, etcetera. I didn't like to be in. Then although I felt ninety per cent better, I kept getting a burning, tearing sensation in my right side where I had the drain. I cannot move when this comes on, I feel faint, light-headed and break out in a sweat. When it goes off, I feel fine. I mentioned it at the six-week check-up and the doctor said it was normal, just part of the healing process. If it isn't any better in the next couple of weeks I shall go to my own doctor. I get so frustrated. Before I felt too ill and exhausted to do anything, now I feel well, but still can't do anything. I shall in time; time is a great healer.

'Any woman who has to have a hysterectomy should have no fears. Women shouldn't listen to anyone who might frighten them, just follow their own instinct. Ask themselves, do I want to be fit or ill? I felt so ill and lifeless I never thought I would ever feel well again. The hysterectomy has taken a lot of strain and stress from out of my life.'


## CHERYL

Cheryl, married but childless, had a total abdominal hysterectomy with removal of one ovary at 31, six months ago. Cheryl had suffered bad stomach pains since the age of 11, but despite investigations no cause was found, and she was accused of 'putting on' the pain. Her periods started at 14 and she began to suffer from migraines. As Cheryl got older, her periods got heavier, lasting twelve days, and the pains continued. Her bowel action was once every seven to ten days. Her GP regulated this with Fybogel and the stomach pains eased a little as well. Cheryl was now 23.

'As my sexual activities progressed I had the coil fitted, which was excellent. I had some pain during intercourse, but put this down to the coil. One day after intercourse

with Mark, now my husband, I was struck with pain in my
side. We were both worried and I went to the doctor. He
did an internal examination and said I had an infection in
my Fallopian tube that would probably make me sterile!
Good bedside manner! He gave me antibiotics.

'Imagine the shock, I had been engaged for three days,
we had known each other four months and hadn't had a
chance to discuss children. I was frightened to lose Mark,
but it was only fair to tell him straight. We had no secrets,
we worked together and he is also my best friend. He was
brilliant and said never mind it's you I want, not what you
can or cannot produce. I was in a health plan at work and
through this I had a laparoscopy, from which they
diagnosed endometriosis. I was 25. I was given
Danazol – 100 mg daily for six months, which stopped my
periods. Up went the weight, intercourse was still painful
and now my side hurt continuously. I'm surprised Mark
married me, but he did the following year.

'I spent the next five years on and off Danazol and had
three laparoscopies, for which I signed agreement for a
hysterectomy, and each time I expected to have one. Mark
and I had discussed hysterectomy and decided that if it
would make me better, to go for it. Mark had come to
terms years before that there would be no children. The
pains were bad and some days the pain in my side would
make me limp. I was continuously tired, cold, had bad
headaches and had put on a lot of weight with the
Danazol. Mark was marvellous, a great support and I
wouldn't have managed without his kindness and
patience.

We moved house and I saw an NHS gynaecologist, for a
second opinion. At the final laparoscopy, they found my
right ovary stuck to my pelvic bone, badly scarred tissue
in and around my womb, and a slight stickiness to my left
ovary. The gynaecologist recommended to have the lot
removed as the condition of my insides gave only a slim
chance of having children. I had to think carefully, the
decision was mine. He put me on the waiting list, while I
did a lot of heart searching. I tried to read up on it, but

there's not much about, especially on my problem and the end result. I went to my GP, but he was useless and said the decision was mine. The sexual side of things did affect our relationship. Mark had always been frightened of hurting me, and most of the time he did. To my surprise, I was called in within a month, so I didn't have much time to think.

'Waking every hour for eight hours to be violently sick was a bad experience after the last laparoscopy. I burst blood vessels in both eyes and under the laparoscopy scar. I had terrible bruising across my belly and underneath so I could hardly walk. I was extremely worried about the hysterectomy, but scared stiff of being sick on coming round from the anaesthetic. The nurses remembered me because of the bruising and Dracula eyes, and said to have a word with the anaesthetist. He said it would probably happen again! I hardly slept with the worry of this and whether it was *the* time to have it all taken away. I awoke with a migraine and cried with fright for most of the morning and made a fool of myself. The other woman in with me had been having flooding sessions and was glad it was all going to be over. The nurses were brilliant and so was everyone else. I'm not usually a cry-baby, I was just scared and anyone else would have been the same, so I'm not ashamed.

'Afterwards I woke to Mark and all was fine with no sickness, I was really pleased. Mark wrote me a letter as I was too busy sleeping, telling me everything went OK. The anaesthetist came to see me twice, he'd read my history and suggested I still had the Danazol in my system at the last laparoscopy and that had caused the after effects. They sent me home on the seventh day. This was much too soon, even though you want to go home. I had no pain-killers or anything, the doctor didn't know I was home, and not even a nurse came to visit.

'I was at home by myself during the day, which I do not recommend. I couldn't have managed without my sister-in-law, who came every day and was brilliant. At the end of the week I went to stay with my parents. *You need someone to look after you all day and night.* Pain is definitely the order of the day and my trusty hot-water bottle was very useful. My bowel movement was a killer, the pain was excruciating and I think I got this as I didn't suffer too badly with wind, like the others. I rang the doctor for help with my motion and found out the pain-killers had constipated me. He advised Paracetamol and laxatives for my bowels.

'Five months later I still had problems with my right side hurting. My GP hoped I hadn't gone through it all for nothing and it wasn't a muscular problem! I nearly throttled him, but the op still needed to be done. I still had headaches and he said until my hormones got working again I'd just have to put up with it.

'Three weeks ago I had the deepest, deepest depression, going into tears at any time. Mark couldn't do anything right. A friend took me to a homeopathic doctor, and I'm glad I went. The doctor listened to me and said I lack calcium and that my hormones weren't working properly. She prescribed one month's homeopathic oestrogen and suggested I have some reflexology. I'm a bit of a sceptic, I'll wait to make my final decision, but I'm feeling quite good. I felt better the next day. I take calcium and Vit E each night as a booster. I also use Vit E as a lubricant for sex, breaking open two capsules and massaging it in. It's marvellous, it's natural and helps to feed the dryness and most of all IT WORKS!!

'The hysterectomy? So much happened leading to the final diagnosis and end results, I'm hoping we made the right decision. I don't think I had much choice, I could imagine myself going back in a year or two to come to the same decision. More heartbreak and ache about kids. So with it not being there at all, it's final. I did see a programme on TV, where a mother had kids for her daughter because she had a hysterectomy after her first-born. They took her eggs and his sperm and placed them both in the mother, *the vessel.* This made me feel a lot better and able to accept my op more. I've got one ovary, Mark has sperm, therefore if we wanted, there's always a

small possibility of us finding a vessel to have kids.
Clutching at straws, but all helps in these early days!!'

## ELLEN

Ellen, a single parent with one son in the Marines, had a
total abdominal hysterectomy with removal of both
ovaries at 41, fifteen months ago.

'I was diagnosed as having severe endometriosis when I
was 21, after complaining of very bad pain from the age of
14 years. I've had many laparoscopies over the years
and hysterectomy was first discussed when I was 29.
At that time I was so desperate to be free of pain, I
said I would go ahead. The gynaecologist then decided not
to operate as I was desperately under weight and he
wasn't happy to remove my ovaries at such a young age. I
was put on the drug Danol, 200 mg three times a day. I
was supposed to be on it for six to nine months, but ended
up taking it for over ten years. There were many bad side
effects, but it did regress my endo until I became very ill
again and had more laparoscopies. I had many adhesions
with endo on my bowel, in the rectum, Pouch of Douglas,
intestines etcetera. No gynaecologist was keen to give me
any major surgery.

'I'd suffered for so long, and had been taking pethidine
daily for pain for eight years. I'd had enough and was at
the "end of my tether"! I found a sympathetic
gynaecologist who was prepared to give me a total
hysterectomy. He *didn't* promise that I would benefit very
much from it, only hoped that I would get some relief. I
fully understood what the operation entailed. I wasn't very
happy about losing both my ovaries, but realized it was
necessary. The gynaecologist said I was "a surgeon's
walking nightmare" as my insides were such a diabolical
mess.

'It took all my courage to go ahead with the
hysterectomy, as I was very frightened. I have many
allergies and had had problems previously after
anaesthesia so I discussed my fears with the anaesthetist

before the op. The op took over five hours, as it was very much worse than first anticipated by the surgeon. I also had bowel surgery since there was endo on my colon. Afterwards, I naturally felt awful, with a lot of post-op pain, infection in the wound, and bladder infections. I had to return to theatre for a cystoscopy (a look inside the bladder) and colonoscopy (a look inside the colon). I was discharged after seven days, much too soon in my opinion, as I was still discharging from both ends of my wound and had a high temperature.

'Things were difficult when I returned home, as I live alone. My son got compassionate leave and did his best to comfort me since I was still very weak and ill. My GP was marvellous, visiting day and night to tend my infected wound. I had hot flushes and night sweats a week after coming home. I was constantly weeping and felt a completely different person to the one I was before. I just didn't feel "me" at all. I got facial shingles, which left me with tri-geminal neuralgia. I had oral thrush, from all the massive doses of antibiotics I was taking for the wound infection.

'I started hormone pills (HRT) for the change, three months after my op, but these made me very sick. I was given skin patches, and was allergic to them with large, red, weeping bumps, and I developed my old endometriosis pain again! A scan showed I had three centimetres of endometriosis in my ovarian sites. It had obviously been microscopic endo which had "fed" on the oestrogens, so HRT was withdrawn. A further pelvic scan three months later showed the endo had regressed, so I can't have any more HRT.

'Fifteen months post-op, it is hell!! I am suffering very severe menopausal symptoms – flushes, sweats, memory loss, bone pain etcetera. At times I do regret having the operation, and I feel in great despair as to how long all this will go on. I get no answers from the medics. Mine is a vicious circle and there seems no answer for me. I worry about osteoporosis and about my cardiovascular system. Apart from the flushes, the nightly sweats and the awful weeping which comes daily, I feel very depressed and sad.

'The positive things are that I won't get ovarian cancer, that I don't need smear tests and I don't have periods. I'd hoped and prayed that the hysterectomy would help me to some extent. Quite honestly I have gained more problems, which are very hard to cope with. I am lucky to have had one baby, I would have liked more, but this was impossible. Endometriosis has ruined my life, my sex life has been non-existent for nineteen years now and I have no desire to resume it at all. The hysterectomy hasn't really made things any easier for me.'

## ROBERTINE

Robertine, married with two grown-up sons, had a total abdominal hysterectomy at the age of 41, twelve months ago. After having a sterilization by laparoscopy, fourteen years ago, Robertine had pains in the scar at the onset of a period. Robertine was living in Holland while this was happening.

'The gynaecologist diagnosed endometriosis (endo) saying there were two ways of curing it – progesterones or hysterectomy. I knew what hysterectomy was and was not shocked. The consultant didn't want to perform a hysterectomy because I was only 28. The doctors in Holland are open and honest, and I had no questions about his reluctance. I wasn't dying, endometriosis was not judged to be a danger, so I was happy enough. I started on a progesterone derivative, which, after trials of different dosages, worked. I had no periods for years and only a slight, dull but continuous pain. Making love got more painful, due to endometriosis and because of a prolapsed uterus. I gained weight and tried all sorts of diets and water retention pills.

'Four years later I had moved to England, which was a culture shock, and I couldn't afford to take time off work and family for surgery. I tried homeopathy which made it all much worse and pains were so bad I usually fainted. I began to get signs of a premature menopause and went back on to another pill, but this didn't help. I went for a second opinion and was told, "Hysterectomy next Saturday, with an HRT implant – you'll feel so much better!!" There just wasn't time for the op. My elder sister also had endo, and was cured after nine months on pills! I tried yet another progesterone unsuccessfully, and ended up on the original pill which seemed to work best of all. I had been travelling to Amsterdam to see my gynaecologist and so transferred to a woman gynaecologist in London.

'Hysterectomy was suggested, but for later, and I stayed on the pills. My life was busy – lorry driving, a nine-hour day in the office, workouts three times a week, lots of walking and a large house to keep clean without any help. Then last year I had a sudden pain at the very bottom of the uterus. The GP said it was a bladder infection and a fibroid and suggested an immediate hysterectomy. It was too sudden, I was confused and anxious that it had all come to a head. I went to the library and got out all the books I could find on hysterectomy, endometriosis and fibroids. I joined the Endometriosis Society and HSG. I saw my consultant who suggested immediate hysterectomy and sent me to another surgeon. He diagnosed adenomyosis and organized a scan. I didn't know what adenomyosis was and looked it up in the library. I also had an explanation from the Endometriosis Society. The scan showed a huge degenerative fibroid, and chocolate cysts. Immediate hysterectomy advised.

'My feelings now cleared, they were not confused or unsure. I had over the years of to-ing and fro-ing got fed up with not being boss over my own body. I had been angry because of the endo, because of the hormones I had to take and because if I forgot to take them, it hurt! My husband was very understanding and supportive. He felt what must be done, should be done. "Lots of work for me, but nasty for her," were his words.

'I had the op the next month in a private hospital and I was happy because of the personal touch. Post-op I felt elated. Everything had gone so smoothly, I hadn't gained any weight and I worked OK, although I did have cystitis and was allergic to the antibiotic used. Once home I felt disappointed that I didn't feel better more quickly. At three months I had had four bladder infections and thrush. At four months I was getting better and had more energy, but was still not the old me yet. It was difficult to cope with normal family problems. I was getting hot flushes and had extreme depression. Blood tests showed severe shortage of oestrogen, but HRT had to wait until the thrush was gone. I have qualms about taking this as my mother has had breast cancer and this is seen as a contraindication of HRT. The gynaecologist and GP have differing views on this, and the gynaecologist says to have a mammogram. It is difficult to find information, but finally I am assured that it has not been proven that HRT causes breast cancer.

'Two swabs showed that the thrush is very deep and severe in bladder, bowel and vagina. I have gained weight and my figure is not what it was. I am angry again, that this has happened to me when I thought it wouldn't. I was in such good shape pre-op. I am angry and impatient about this wretched thrush and will do anything to stop it. My husband finds the thrush a pain in the penis! Tiresome and bothersome, he will do all he can to clear it and feels, "how awful for her". I am also angry that after all I've been through I might have to take yet another pill for the rest of my life to suppress the menopause symptoms.

'Six months post-op I'm having no serious menopausal symptoms. I'm not sleeping well, but I'm not taking drugs for it. I am frustrated about the weight on the thighs and tum after all the effort of losing it. I'm very tired at times, but am working full-time again. I cannot physically do as much as I used to and am very forgetful. I'm angry and disappointed at the length of recovery time, but on the whole pleased I had it done.

'Gradually I found I was very depressed and having difficulties coping at home. Unlike me, I became tearful and dissatisfied with my life. I quit my job as partner of our family business. My gynaecologist finally convinced me that my depressions were due to the menopause. She and my GP are both confident for me to have HRT as the risk of cancer is so slight, despite my mother's history. Now a year post-op, I have had HRT for two months and feel *much* better, almost back to my normal, happy self. I have the occasional, severe headache, but these are expected to go after about three months of HRT. The thrush problem has been solved for both of us, but the excess weight will not go without yet another diet. I have a new job after being "headhunted" by a major insurance company to train as a financial consultant. I'm weight-lifting again and have started singing lessons.'

## APRIL

April, married for the second time, with three children from her first marriage, had a total abdominal hysterectomy at 42, four years ago. April has experienced pain on ovulation since her periods started at 12. Following termination of pregnancy and sterilization by laparoscopy, ten years ago, April's periods became very painful and heavy. Later that year, she received laser treatment for a cervical lesion. April has a chronic back problem.

'I was advised that the heavy, painful periods were due to emotional causes!! I could have a hysterectomy if I wanted one. I was appalled and rejected the idea, as I didn't feel there was enough wrong with me to warrant such a drastic operation at 32.

'My periods were painful and prolonged with clots and flooding. Nine years later I had a D and C and a laparoscopy after emergency admission to hospital for pain, and was advised to have a hysterectomy. I was training to be a social worker and it was inconvenient to have the op. I accepted that I would probably end up having the operation, and felt slightly troubled by this, but didn't have time to think about it. Two years later, I was again admitted as an emergency, after pain and bleeding between periods. I was told of a lump which could be a twisted ovary, or ovarian cyst and/or a malignancy. I had discovered the lump when I'd felt the painful area in my side and found it under the skin. I knew, then, something was wrong, but forgot about it for a few weeks. I was advised to consider, most carefully, having a hysterectomy soon. I was resigned to the idea since I knew I couldn't go on as I was. Not only were my periods now a social embarrassment at times, highly inconvenient and painful, but I was feeling ill. I talked it over with my partner and we discussed it together with my consultant, who explained everything I wanted to know. He included my partner and warned him how I might be following the operation, emphasizing what I shouldn't do.

'I read a lot about the operation and contacted HSG. I was afraid I'd be depressed post-op and that my back would be troublesome. I was terrified of being sick afterwards as I usually am. The anaesthetist assured me he'd make a "mix" and post-op, I wasn't sick, just a bit nauseous. My back was hell for two days and I had to be turned every hour, day and night. I think, on the whole, it's been made worse by the op.

'I had the op privately. I had adenomyosis, multiple fibroids – one as big as a baby's head – cervicitis, adhesions, and the appendix stuck to one Fallopian tube. I didn't know what adenomyosis was and looked it up in the library.

'I had a lot of post-op pain and had to contend with a lot of noise and undue disturbances. The window cleaner and noisy workmen actually came into my room to work at one stage!! Most significantly upsetting was a baby crying constantly. It all added up to a stressful experience. Not a good private hospital at all. The consultant and nurses were most apologetic, kind and caring. However "matron" came to see me about my complaints of excessive noise, dirty room, awful food and the disturbances, and inferred that I was "upset" by the op. I was furious, and also began to feel anxious and rather afraid after this, and I felt profound relief to be discharged on the sixth day.

'At home I experienced confusion and disorientation. It was a real effort to be articulate, and I couldn't think or write properly; it took me ages to write a few sentences. Noises sounded exceedingly loud and I felt giddy all the time. I had very little desire to eat and lost weight. I found people difficult to cope with and just wanted to be left alone. I lacked concentration and was devastatingly tired. I hadn't been told to expect any of this and I was grateful for the support of HSG, then, as I thought I was going crazy at one point! I was short-tempered and weepy, with "good and bad" days, but being forewarned by the consultant helped me cope with this. My partner was understanding and caring all the way through and stayed home for three weeks to look after me. He was very supportive, but didn't seem able to cope with my confusion and just didn't understand it. He accepted me having the operation, totally, his concern being for my health, and he knew the op would benefit me. He is a naturally caring man. I felt relief that I could look forward to a pain-free life that wasn't controlled by my periods and was glad I'd had the op. I was upset by all the problems I'd experienced and hadn't read, or been told about. I feel that but for the support I received there's a possibility I'd have been a "psychological" case.

'Sex wasn't a problem. We resumed intercourse just before the consultant had advised we should. At first I felt a bit nervous and tender, but the only after effect I've noticed since the op, is that orgasm is less intense and briefer.

'When I felt able to cope I wrote and complained to the hospital about my in-patient stay. Correspondence flowed back and forth for a while, but eventually fizzled out. I was left without redress, feeling upset and angry at being labelled "upset by the operation and reacting emotionally to it". I was further devastated by the enforced inactivity and became demoralized, very bored and subsequently depressed. I was incredibly clumsy and was staggeringly tired. I had night sweats. I felt a sense of loss and cried a lot. I had a mental image, for a while, of having a hole in my abdomen where my womb should be. I was surprised by this in view of all the preparatory reading I'd done. I went through a grieving process for a few weeks.

'I was upset when I painfully ovulated and had an acute sense of having had the op in vain!! Three months post-op, my young, male GP brushed aside my feelings of tiredness, saying I'd feel better when I returned to work and a "normal" routine. I mentioned having a scan for the ovulation problem and he didn't like that. The consultant had examined my ovaries and found nothing wrong and how did I know it was ovulation pain?!! I suggested the possibility of hormone treatment and he said he only knew of the pill and I was too old for that. I felt I'd been slapped in the face and went home and cried. I felt old and useless. I got angry and changed my GP to a woman doctor, who suggested pain-killers or an oopherectomy, which I refused. She said that my age was against me regarding taking the pill. My consultant had a "wait and see" attitude and still hadn't done anything six months later. He refused to prescribe HRT, even to prevent osteoporosis, which my mother has.

'I went to see a leading specialist on HRT who gave me an oestrogen/testosterone implant. The testosterone caused hair growth on my legs and an exaggerated libido, which caused such problems between my husband and I that we went to Marriage Guidance (Relate). This proved very useful, as it revealed that my husband was reacting to the hysterectomy after all. Although he's never wanted children of his own, he subconsciously felt a sense of loss over me no longer being able to carry his child. My sex drive had always been stronger than his and he felt very threatened by mine being further increased, and couldn't cope with it. This all became a bigger issue in one sense, as I'd applied to become a Marriage Guidance counsellor and my application was turned down as I was going for counselling myself. I felt very angry with my husband over this. By this time I was involved with a voluntary group (HSG) and feel it was a good thing that I was doing something useful and helping other women. The testosterone was stopped and our sexual problems have subsequently lessened.

'The op had good and bad effects. I'm totally glad I had it and revel in being able to plan my life without worrying about pain and bleeding. Rather like men, who take this "freedom" for granted! I'm sad about all the post-op problems and that the op didn't help the ovulation problem. I feel I suffered a lot unnecessarily, because of things out of my direct control. I was not "listened to" by my GP or consultant and feel my recovery was hindered by a lot of things that could have been avoided. I'm sad that the op had such far-reaching and unexpected effects upon my marriage. However these, like my scar, have now faded away!'

## SARA

Sara, married with two boys 13 and 10 years old, had a total abdominal hysterectomy at 39, a year ago. Sara is self-employed as a peripatetic music teacher which involves a lot of driving and is a busy, demanding job. Sara had back problems during her pregnancies, due to 'a bit of something missing' in her back.

'I'd always had problems with very heavy bleeding and bad period pains, except when on the pill. Two years prior to the op the pains and bleeding got worse causing such tiredness. Even though I had several D and Cs, nothing changed. When I agreed to have a hysterectomy, I understood what the operation meant, but it bothered me a great deal that I would be convalescing for twelve weeks. Friends warned me that I would be unable to do anything when I first got home. I felt quite hysterical at times during the two months I was waiting to go in. I had no relatives nearby to help with washing, shopping and cooking. The thought of "walking out" on my husband and sons for ten days and needing help on my return was quite appalling. I very nearly cancelled the whole thing, only common sense made me walk into the hospital and go through with it. I had adenomyosis. My husband thought the hysterectomy was a good idea and supported me all the way through the trauma of getting ready, being in hospital and convalescence. I had been previously sterilized and that did mean we had already decided, no more children, so I didn't have that problem to worry about. Being self-employed, I had to organize everything for my period of absence as well as stock the house up with food. I became very tired prior to the op.

'I made good progress after the op in hospital, but a week after coming home had an abdominal infection. Fortunately I'm married to a very patient, supportive and loving husband who took nearly three weeks off to handle the situation. My sons also rallied round admirably, as did a few friends. Normally a very active person, I found recovery slow. I was used to dashing here, there and everywhere, playing "beat the clock". I was driving short distances at six weeks and doing light household duties and my consultant said I could go back to work at seven weeks. I didn't go back, as I couldn't drive far enough and had difficulty standing for any length of time. I needed to spend two hours a day flat on my back in order to reduce backache and lower abdominal ache. I had pushed myself forward, but still felt mentally and physically tired.

'I felt guilty not returning to work as the consultant said I should and also because my mother and some friends seemed very surprised that I was tired and still needed to lie down. My mother had a hysterectomy thirty years ago and can't remember any pain or tiredness at all! My back was a problem and no one, consultant, GP or hospital, suggested anything for it. I needed to take life slower and to have time to lie down, so I delayed returning to work until three months post-op. I found it tiring for the first month, but then felt better and by six months the tiredness was gone and I felt fully recovered.

'Two things I found helpful. Stocking up the freezer pre-op with casseroles, and doing what my body told me really worked for me. There has been no difference in our sex life. Nine months post-op I returned from the first "gynae" – free holiday I'd had for a long time. It was great. A year later I am really noticing the benefits of hysterectomy.'

# 5.
# CANCER OF THE WOMB

Although younger women are susceptible, cancer of the womb occurs mainly in older women, when heavy, irregular bleeding around the time of the change is quite often the first sign that something is wrong. It is not usually apparent from a cervical smear which gives information only about the cervix. However, occasionally the spread of the cancer may produce irregularities in the cervix that are picked up either at the examination prior to the smear being taken or on the Pap smear. This was how cancer was detected in the very young, childless woman of 26 in this chapter. The other three women are married with children and aged between 41 and 60, one of whom had a radical hysterectomy and radium treatment. There has never been any link between sexual intercourse, promiscuity and cancer of the womb. There is little choice about having a hysterectomy in these circumstances.

## AMY

Amy, married with two grown-up children, had a total abdominal hysterectomy with removal of both ovaries at 50, seven years ago. Amy has asthma but otherwise had been quite well until the year before her op. Her demanding full-time job was as an executive with a nationwide company and involved driving.

'When I was 49 I began to get very heavy, almost continuous bleeding. I went to my GP, who said it was my age, but agreed to give me a smear test. I was shown the result, normal cells only, and it was all clear. I asked again about the bleeding and was again told it was my age and would stop in time. It still hadn't stopped seven months later so I asked to see a gynaecologist. My GP agreed and two months later, I saw the hospital doctor and a D and C was arranged. After the D and C the doctor said I could go home, but would I return on Monday to see the consultant, who would want to do a hysterectomy and/or Deep X-Ray Treatment (DXT). I asked if I had cancer as I wanted to know, and was told that I did! I was shocked, deeply shocked, as I had believed my GP that the bleeding was due to my age. I didn't want anyone to see how shocked and upset I was and went to the bathroom and cried. My first reaction was: "What a shame, I'm going to die, I won't see my boys married." I couldn't believe this was really happening to me. That weekend at home I kept thinking about the cancer and breaking down and feeling very unhappy.

'My husband came with me to see the lady consultant, who confirmed that I needed a total hysterectomy and removal of my ovaries. It didn't dawn on me what was going to happen, I'd never thought I'd have a hysterectomy. I didn't know very much apart from the fact that I was losing my womb, which was the cause of the bleeding, and my ovaries. I found out some information from HSG, and the gynaecologist was very helpful, but when something comes as a shock, it doesn't sink in. I went into hospital the next month.

'I thought the op went well, as I wasn't as wheezy with asthma as I had been after the D and C. I wasn't given any information unless I asked for it and so I asked. I was told I could drive after four weeks, I wasn't to do much lifting, my return to work was up to my GP and I could go home after ten days. I had no trouble after the op in hospital.

'For the first week or so I thought about the cancer a lot, but felt as they had taken the womb away, which was an entire organ, it should be all right. The next few weeks I felt unhappy a couple of times a day, but I kept thinking they've taken it away, and I haven't had DXT so maybe I wasn't going to need it. At the post-op check I was told that they had caught the cancer in time and I wouldn't be having DXT. I got over the op very quickly and was back to work in two months. It was too soon, but it was my choice and I won a trip to America, which I'll always remember. I didn't lift anything and I drove very carefully. I thought about the cancer once or twice a day, but then found some days I hadn't thought about it at all. After that I was very busy working and it would be a week or so before I thought. Now I never think about it unless I hear of someone else who has the same. My family, of course, were worried and concerned for me. Following on from my op, so many close members of the family were ill and needed me, us, to look after them, that really we just had to get on with what lay ahead. We had four family deaths within a short time, three were our parents and for whom we mourned deeply.

'During the first year, I experienced all the symptoms of the menopause, hot sweats etcetera, as I could not have HRT. This was rather tiresome at times, but really I didn't have time to dwell on it; I kept very busy. We did resume sex, but there were a few problems for me with a dry, sore, itchy vagina. I was given creams for this, but these didn't help. After about a year, I saw my gynaecologist and she sent me for a blood sugar test for diabetes. It was found I had diabetes (this was the cause of my problem) and needed treatment. I have a high vaginal vault smear for cancer when I go for my yearly check-up.

'Looking back, I feel again how deeply shocked I was; it had never entered my head for a moment that I had cancer. Now I never think of it and I'm just glad to be alive. I've seen one son married and I enjoy being a grandma. I never worry about cancer or the hysterectomy, which saved my life. In fact I've worried far more about the brain op (not connected to cancer) I've had since than anything else.'

## EMMA

Emma, married, with a grown-up family, had a radical hysterectomy with removal of cervix, womb, both ovaries and the top third of her vagina, after two treatments of radium, at 60, four years ago. Emma has a history of cancers of the salivary gland and breast, both of which were successfully treated. Emma also suffers with high blood pressure. She is completely deaf.

'I was still having regular periods at the age of 59, when they became more frequent and I was bleeding non-stop. This lasted for six months and I went into hospital for a D and C. I was rather tense about going in, as I am totally deaf. Several other women were in for the same thing and I quite enjoyed "chatting" to them, armed with my notepad! We were told we would be in for three days and one by one they went home, but not me! The nurses couldn't tell me anything, just that I would see the doctor at the end of the week. On that day I was in a state of anxiety, as I had a premonition that something was very wrong. As I walked into the office, the lady doctor looked over her glasses and said: "I am sorry to tell you this, but you have cancer of the uterus." I was in a state of shock, I could not take it in, I felt numb. She thought it was contained in the womb, and that they might catch it in time, but I would have to have a hysterectomy, after deep radium treatment (DRT).

'My son was waiting for me outside and when I told him, he broke down. He cried and held me tight, but strangely I felt quite calm and it was me who was doing the comforting! There was no question of not having it done, it was a matter of life or death.

'I returned to hospital for the DRT and went down to theatre. When I came back to a steel-lined room, I was hooked up to the radium equipment, wires and a cable running up between my legs into the vagina. The machine was at the bottom of the bed, I had a catheter in and tablets to constipate me. I couldn't move and this lasted several days until they came to take it out. Not very pleasant! The worst bit was when they told me to push hard as if I was having a baby and everything came out in a rush, padding, cotton wool, wires and all the horrible muck! I went back a month later for another session. My consultant believed in DRT *before* the operation, instead of after, as this gave me a better chance.

'The next month I went in for my hysterectomy. I was worried about the anaesthetic because of the blood pressure. I had lots of tests before going down, but I felt a bit nervous as I was deaf and didn't know what was going on. Everyone was very kind and understanding and wrote things down for me, which helped enormously. I wanted a bikini cut as I had heard it didn't show so much, but it was up to the surgeon. When I came round I'd had my wish, a bikini cut. Everything was taken, and a third of my vagina, so it is very short. I had a catheter in and when they came to take it out, it wouldn't come. It was awful, everyone tugging like mad and I was hitting the ceiling, before they finally removed it. It is very rare for that to happen.

'The hospital sent me away for two weeks convalescence and it was lovely, I didn't want to come home! All of us women had the same op and we used to hobble, holding our tums, to the village coffee shop. We all bought track suits to wear from the village shop and the villagers called us the "crippled crumpet"!

'Where I was stitched in the vagina is still a bit painful, as the skin is very thin due to the radium. When I go for my check-ups and internal examination, it always hurts when they reach the top. They have given me hormone cream, which helps a little, but I am not allowed HRT because of my cancer history. I get attacks of cystitis and have had a cystoscopy and dilatation of the bladder, hoping it would cure it, but it hasn't. My gynaecologist thinks it is due to the DRT I had before surgery. Otherwise I don't really feel any different. I am fairly fit, went cycling last year on holiday, do my exercises, sit-ups etcetera. I have a job as a secretary/assistant and I rarely think about the fact that I have had a hysterectomy. As for the benefit, that speaks for itself. I was cured of cancer.'

## SHELLEY

Shelley, single, but in a long-term relationship, with no children, had a total abdominal hysterectomy at 26, five months ago. About eighteen months previously Shelley had a termination of pregnancy.

'Six months ago I went to a clinic for my two-yearly cervical smear. The doctor noticed peculiarities and called in the head of the unit. I was referred to the nearby hospital with an appointment for that very afternoon. I had thought the day would just be routine, see you next year sort of thing. I was shocked and cried hysterically. At the hospital, it was confirmed that something was abnormal. Strange how in the morning I was quite shy, but now I didn't care who had a look. I was booked in for a cone biopsy two days later. They certainly were moving fast which made me suspect something was seriously wrong. The doctor said he suspected nothing "sinister" and that under general anaesthetic he would check my bladder.

'After the cone biopsy, I had slight bleeding and terrible pains, needing a lot of pain-killers. I lost a lot of brown yuck over the next couple of weeks and wrote in my diary "I wish I felt 100 per cent better". I was depressed. Then I woke up in a pool of bright red blood and D, my chap, took me to hospital, where it stopped and I was told to rest. A week later a letter arrived and D came to the office and read it to me. "I regret to inform you . . ." I felt very weak, my wrists and ankles felt strange.

'I never wanted kids, but it's funny how you do when you know you can't. I think I always did want them really, it was just a career-minded smart thing to say. I was hurt, but the people around me were devastated. I felt guilty, especially towards D, who had always wanted a family. The first thing he said was "What have I got to look forward to in old age?" It was an off-the-cuff remark, a bit like someone saying something when they're drunk, which they regret later, but it is their true feeling. I knew then I would never marry D, I would never tie him to me, though we would continue to live together. I pushed him away a bit; I felt alone. I'd always thought I was aware of my body and I really felt I had let myself down. The most nagging doubt, Why me? It's associated with loose women and I felt dirty. D also felt guilty and wondered if in some way he had given it to me. I hoped all my friends would have ugly deformed children that would keep them poor, while I lived like a film star. I had some nice antiques; I wondered who I would leave them to. I was 26 years old and really thought I was going to die. I thought, All this is over, when really it hadn't even started.

'The gynaecologist, who explained in detail how the cancer had travelled, saw us together. Radiotherapy was not a good alternative as it would age my vagina, shrivel it up and sex would be painful. My life was in danger, I had to have a hysterectomy, hopefully further treatment post-op would not be necessary. The doctor spent a long time with us and was willing to spend more if need be.

'I'd always associated hysterectomy with sterilization, or a cure for terrible period pains in older women, never with someone like me. I expected to gain weight, lose my waist and prematurely age. I felt isolated, as if I was the first person to have this at my age. My friends brought me books, which though they explained procedures, still made me feel unique. D was angry at me reading the books, he felt they depressed me. They did in a way, but I was determined to know it all. I had let my body down once and I wasn't going to do it again. I didn't care about the scar, my main fear was the anaesthetic. I would be out for four hours and I imagined I wouldn't wake up. Should I write a will? Would everyone be upset when I died? Would my mother ever get over my death? I felt very morbid.

'I went into hospital just a month after the smear, everything had happened so fast! For the X-rays I had to lie still with a belt around my middle for twenty minutes. I felt fidgety and cried. D was brought in to calm me, but it didn't work. I cried in bed that night, I couldn't sleep and my mind was working overtime. I was allowed out the day before the op and D and I had lunch together. I felt very close to him, we have been going out together for five years and I still love him to bits. Back in hospital I felt tired and irritable and when the visitors left, depressed. The next day I cried the whole journey to theatre. I decided that there is no such thing as God and if there was he would hardly do this to me. I felt he would punish me for thinking that and I was probably going through this now because of something in my past. Just before my injection I made them promise to leave my ovaries. I think everyone I knew was looking at their watches and lived through it with me.

'I did not believe they had taken my womb away, I was convinced they'd opened me up, looked, decided it was okay and sewn me back up again. I couldn't see my scar, my stomach was so swollen, and I laughed at the pink antiseptic paint plastered on me. It looked like I was wearing boxer shorts. I had drips everywhere, but the worst thing was the wind pain! I had survived the anaesthetic, now I wanted to survive the wind pain. Everyone seemed thrilled about my scar and how I'd still be able to wear a bikini, but I'd never worn a bikini in my life. Then I got the all-clear, the cancer had been contained in the womb! I should have been ecstatic, but wondered if the op had been absolutely necessary. I cried a lot that day. The hardest thing to come to terms with is the feeling of guilt to my own body.

'At home D wanted it all out in the open, to make me face it, but it didn't help me very much. The issue of children doesn't exist yet as far as I'm concerned, I'll face that later, first I want to feel 100 per cent. The top of the vagina has not knit exactly and I am back to the hospital every three weeks or so. It is better than it was. I am not bleeding and sex is not quite so sore, but I've not had regular sex yet. I am a bit scared of it. D is very good, he feels a bit neglected, but doesn't want to hurt me. He is a bit wary too. We have had our problems, but I hope we are over the worst.

'My friends have been amazing and have come through when it counts, and I am closer to my family, who felt they might lose me. The only bad patch has been with D. I feel I have let him down, although he says he wants me, not a baby-making machine. I kept pushing him away, but it was my guilt; I felt I had deprived him of something. It was as gruelling for him as it was for me, but in a different way. He has proved to be a real treasure. I have not felt depressed, but I'm shocked at all the evil thoughts I had pre-op. Everything seems geared to children, yet I know they cause heartache. I could always adopt, although I doubt I will. I feel much more attached to my godson. I wonder that I will never go through childbirth, or breast feeding and wonder what it is like. I feel I am depriving both our parents of grandchildren. I stop all this defeatism by remembering we are shaped by our experience in life and I do believe I am a stronger person for all of this. I have had to come to terms with why I am working so hard, who will reap the reward. I now know I am working for myself; my responsibilities are to myself, D and the mortgage. I wonder who will take care of me when I am an old lady, but it's probably worse to be an old lady neglected by your children. I guess I am still sad about what has happened. If I had my time over again, I would have a child earlier when I had the chance.'

## MILLIE

Millie, married for the second time with two married sons from her first marriage, had a total abdominal hysterectomy and removal of both ovaries at 41, four years ago. Her second husband, Harry, had a chronic heart condition that required constant medical supervision and meant he was restricted to a wheelchair outside the home.

'My monthlies had sort of dribbled away by the time I was thirty-eight, that was the year I got married again. Following that I lost a bit now and again on odd days or had just a smear on my pants. I was never one for the sex side of marriage and hadn't had any since before my first husband died. Harry's not well enough for anything like that. Then I started to bleed really heavy, fresh blood. Harry was often in hospital and I didn't say anything to him when he was home, but he just seemed to know after a while. He kept on that I should go to the doctor, but I didn't. I never had a smear or anything like that and I didn't like the thought of it. I just got on with things. I never mentioned it to the boys or their wives. I didn't see much of them anyway.

'I had another big bleed and was very weak and Harry called my doctor home. Really I suppose I was pleased he did. The doctor was new, very nice and kind, I hadn't seen him before and he sent me to hospital. I had a lot of tests and some blood. I was glad of the rest as I had been feeling ill and needed sleep. They said I would need a hysterectomy and I thought, well they know best. I wasn't sure what it was about, but I didn't like to bother the nurses, they were so busy. Some of the other ladies had had one and I talked to them. I don't like operations, but I knew I had something bad. You just know these things, but I couldn't just go in like that for a long time, as Harry was at home. I was worried about him, he was waiting to go into hospital, too, for an operation. He couldn't get up to see me and the boys wouldn't bring him. They were upset that I was ill and hadn't told them and I think they blamed it on Harry.

'I went back into hospital six weeks later and at the same time Harry was admitted. The nurses were lovely and brought him to see me a couple of times. He was worried; as he couldn't do anything for me, he thought the op was probably the best thing. Well I couldn't go on the way I was. The doctors and nurses were all very nice and did a lot for me. One doctor came and had a chat and asked if I had anything I was worried about. He said I was very ill and it was major surgery.

'I was glad when it was over. I found the thought of the anaesthetic really played on my mind this time. I had loads of tubes and things all over the place! When I had my stitches out I didn't heal very well, my wound leaked

and gaped really badly. I was in hospital three weeks till it
was better. They told me I had a cancer of the womb and
they had taken everything, my ovaries as well, so it had
been bad. I wasn't so upset really. I think both Harry and
I knew it was cancer.

'It has taken a lot out of me, and I should have done
something in the beginning, but there didn't seem to be the
time and I didn't have the "go" to face it. I'm really
grateful to the doctors and nurses, they did so much and
helped me such a lot. The hysterectomy as such, didn't
worry me, but the whole thing of going into hospital and
needing all that treatment! That was something I'd never
dreamed of and if I'd known I don't know that I could've
managed it. Getting well is taking a long time, I'm still
poorly and under hospital supervision.

'The boys never got over how ill I was and somehow
they do blame Harry. It is strange, they used to be so
close; Harry was an uncle to them for years, even before
their dad died. They come and see me more now, not long
visits, but they hardly say a word to Harry. I've now got
two grandchildren, I never thought I'd live to see any, and
I'm so happy to see them. I think the hysterectomy has
given me a bit more time and I thank God for that.'

# 6.
# CANCER OF THE CERVIX

This is the one cancer that has a detectable pre-cancer stage allowing treatment to prevent further development. The cervical smear test has a high detection rate, but mainly of cancer and pre-cancerous cells in the cervix, nowhere else. The pre-cancer cell was seen as slow-growing, taking many years to become cervical cancer. Most (80 per cent) cases were found in women over 40, but in recent years there has been a steady increase in the number of cases detected in women under 35.

Cervical cancer currently carries a lot of emotional baggage due to the reported link between its occurrence and sexual intercourse. It is not true that cervical cancer is a sign of promiscuity, and as experienced by one of the women in this chapter, there are causes totally unrelated to the sexual experience. Of the four women in this chapter, only one is over 40, one is single and two have children. Three had a radical hysterectomy, two with follow-up radiotherapy. Although some women have a hysterectomy for three or more 'abnormal' smear results showing pre-cancer cells, all the women here were diagnosed as having cancer.

## JOANNE

Joanne, married with two children, had a Wertheim's hysterectomy with removal of womb, cervix, top third of vagina and lymph nodes, three years ago. This was followed by radiotherapy. Joanne was 32.

'Four years ago I went to my doctor because I was experiencing bleeding when I had intercourse. The female locum took a smear, said I had an erosion and sent off for a hospital appointment. A few weeks later I was told there was "much pus" on the smear and it should be repeated in three to six months time. I thought it must be an infection and wasn't worried. The hospital appointment came and I rang to see if it would be worth going as I was pregnant. The sister in charge of the clinic said not to come, but to tell the doctor at my ante-natal appointment. I did and no one seemed concerned, after all erosions often cleared up after pregnancy. I asked for a repeat smear when I was five months pregnant, but my slightly deaf doctor didn't hear me. He was so busy, I didn't like to make a fuss.

'I had intermittent bleeding again and the doctor confirmed it was a threatened miscarriage. It was pretty difficult to rest with a 2-year-old to look after and I asked for the erosion to be checked; if the bleeding was due to that, I wouldn't have to keep resting. There was no sign of the erosion and this should have been a relief, but left me worrying about what was causing the spotting. Eventually I stopped saying anything, but I was puzzled and concerned.

'My baby was a week overdue and I carefully felt my cervix. I'd had the coil before so knew what I felt like inside. I knew that the cervix was supposed to soften if labour was imminent, but it was hard and *lumpy*! This did worry me and the worst thing, I couldn't tell anybody. How could I say that I had felt inside myself! I can say it now, but I still feel that somehow I shouldn't have. I gave birth to a beautiful baby girl and everything was wonderful. A few weeks later I checked my cervix and decided, as it felt the same, I would ask for a repeat smear at my six-week post-natal check. The doctor sent for me before then as the lab had written to ask why I hadn't been back. I was very relieved that I was going to get a repeat smear, I just knew something wasn't right. My doctor did the smear and said that I had "polyps" (nodules of tissue on short stalks) that must be sorted out straightaway and I wasn't to worry if the hospital got in touch very quickly. I was relieved that something was being done, but was surprised to hear from the hospital that very afternoon with an appointment for two days later.

'My husband and children came with me to the hospital and a biopsy was arranged for the next week. The consultant said we weren't to worry and mentioned my earlier smear had shown "abnormal cells". This was the first I knew of this! Strangely I wasn't really worried. I vaguely knew what a biopsy was for, but something seemed to stop the knowledge coming to the front of my mind. There seemed to be a switch-off mechanism inside me. I was being looked after, worrying wouldn't change anything and they wouldn't find anything serious. The baby came in with me for the biopsy, as I was breast-feeding. The results would take a week. I was told not to worry and again I didn't, there was going to be nothing wrong! All I listened to was "Don't worry", and the fact that he had removed a *large* lump from the back of the cervix barely registered. The switch-off mechanism was in operation.

'The results. I just burst into tears when the consultant said I had invasive cervical cancer and would need a radical hysterectomy, with removal of lymph nodes. He hoped that further treatment would not be necessary. He looked surprised that I was crying and said that surely I had known something was wrong!! I remember wondering what on earth he expected me to do! At that moment I was in complete shock. The word cancer overrode everything else – I might die! I realized that that was it! No more children. I was pleased I had my two girls which was a combination I had always wanted, and I felt relieved that they weren't going to remove my ovaries so I wouldn't have an early menopause.

'I wanted to take the baby in with me again, but the consultant explained that there weren't the facilities for this. Also I would be quite unwell and with all the drugs, radio-active chemicals for X-rays and body scans, it would be better to stop breast-feeding. I had five days in which to stop and was helped by a good friend in the National

Childbirth Trust (NCT), but the shock really stopped the milk. At the time the significance of a hysterectomy didn't really hit home. I didn't know if I'd be around that long to worry about it. I was quite apprehensive about the actual operation and the aftermath. My mother gave me the benefit of her experience, telling me I would have terrible wind pains afterwards and need peppermint cocktails.

'On the day of the op, the anaesthetist offered me tranquillizers before the pre-med and I took what he offered and went to theatre as high as a kite. My ovaries had been left. I went home after nine days, having been told that I mustn't lift anything!! I had to look after and lift my 6-week-old baby. Then I needed radiotherapy, which stopped my ovaries functioning anyway. It really took it out of me and I didn't have the energy for playing, etcetera, with the children. However, friends and family were marvellous and we were soon over the worst.

'It was then that it began to hit me. I was different from all my friends, how would I feel visiting them when they had babies? How would I feel if they complained of PMT? Did they think I was different? I felt very alone and I did feel different. I had always thought that I would feel a bit useless when I wasn't able to have children any more and now it had happened. I was no longer a productive member of the human race. It sounds crazy, but I had to give it a lot of thought before I could feel okay about it. What if the children wanted a baby, how would I cope with my feelings? Was it fair on my husband and worst of all, what if something happened to the girls? I felt I would want to die, it would be unjust and unbearable. Not that children can be replaced, but I didn't even have that choice any more. My way of coping with all this pain was to recite a little formula every time I started to feel bad and wanted to cry:

1) Really I could only cope properly with two children.
2) I didn't have to worry about contraception.
3) I didn't have periods, every woman's dream.

Deep inside I was grieving for that part of myself that I

had lost. It felt so hopeless, crying certainly wouldn't change it and it was silly to waste time crying. Between four to eighteen months post-op, I felt upset that I had had to have a hysterectomy, it had nothing to do with the cancer. I felt life was unfair and why me?

'Three years later I really don't think about it all that much. I am happy with my family and am glad I can't be tempted to have another child. I am still a woman and have discovered a lot of new things. I have more faith in myself and more self-esteem now. This is partly a result of having cancer. I've had a scare and been given a second chance to make more of life. Partly as a result of the hysterectomy, I know I have more to offer than the fact that I can have children; there is more to me than that! I still feel sad sometimes and I don't like having to take hormones every day, but the long-term effects are positive. My remaining fear is what would I do if something happened to the girls, but that is crazy because there's no way another baby could compensate for that anyway.'

## CORINYA

Corinya, single and childless, had a radical hysterectomy with removal of womb, cervix, top third of vagina and lymph nodes, two years ago. Corinya was 27, her only family is a married brother living some distance away.

'I'd had several boyfriends, but only one sexual partnership, when I lived with a boyfriend for four years. This ended two years before the op, mainly because of my very demanding job as a rep and the career opportunities that came my way. I had never had any problems with my periods and had always had regular smears. A smear came back with a positive result and I was told to return for another in six months. This worried me and I went to a private specialist for a second opinion. An excellent doctor, he did a colposcopy and told me I had invasive cancer of the cervix and advised a radical hysterectomy. I was shocked, I hadn't actually expected cancer. I went in for the op very quickly, under the NHS, and everyone was very kind and gentle. I was numb and amazed at the speed of it all and that it had happened to me.

'I was discharged home after ten days, having been told that I wouldn't need further treatment, they had got it all. A close friend came and stayed for a couple of weeks, but then I was on my own. I recovered physically quite quickly; I was determined to get back to work and to being normal as soon as possible. I was working, part-time, by eight weeks, feeling dreadfully tired, but determined. I was still numb and rather uptight, especially over the social inference that only promiscuous women got cancer of the cervix. It seemed dreadfully unfair to go through all that I had, and then be condemned out of hand. I didn't talk to anyone, not even my brother, about what I'd had done or what it was for.

'I began to realize that the second opinion had probably saved my life. Around three months post-op I went to a discussion group of women who'd had a hysterectomy. There were two older women who'd had the same as me, but not such radical surgery. I was amazed at how similar my feelings were to those voiced, although I sat silent through the whole session. Suddenly it hit me how angry I was, dreadfully angry. I needed to talk to someone, to work through the shock and insanity of it all. Not as one in a group, but on a one-to-one basis, to understand the meaning of it all for me and why it had happened. I spoke many times with a lovely lady from HSG; I was no nearer understanding it all, but talking helped.

'I returned for a hospital check and high vaginal smear, this came back positive. I was shocked again, but into anger. No one had said that cancer of the cervix could grow in the vagina or the perineum. Okay, the very fact that one continues to have smears should have meant something, but it didn't. I felt betrayed and very, very frightened. How could it return? I'd not had a sexual partner for over two years. What chance was there for me if it had returned? I had laser beam treatment to the vagina. I was told it wouldn't hurt, but it was excruciatingly painful. I needed to talk to the doctors, but they didn't answer my questions.

'My next smear was clear, but then I had a swelling in my groin and pain in the leg on that side, and some days, difficulty walking. I desperately rang round for someone to talk to, nurses, doctors; I was feeling very angry. Why me? What was happening here? Why wouldn't anyone talk to me about what was happening to *my* body? It was my life trickling away. At the clinic I was told the lump was a suspicious cyst, and they would do a biopsy. I still didn't get any answers to my questions.

'The biopsy result was confusing, part being negative, part questionable and I was given radiotherapy, but this was useless, the cyst grew larger. I didn't get on with the doctor, who also wouldn't make time to talk to me. I behaved rather badly one day, letting it all out screaming, shouting and crying. The nurse asked if I was all right? Stupid question! I told her no and she went and got sister and they stood there looking at me, before suggesting I talk to the doctor! I walked off and gatecrashed the gynaecologist's clinic. I hadn't seen him for months and he was like balm to my wounded spirit. He listened as I ranted and raved a bit and then spat out my fears about the "cyst" getting larger. He gave me time and in doing that, he gave me much more, and I began to feel I really mattered after all.

'I started chemotherapy which was totally awful and difficult to persevere with, but I didn't lose my hair. Each treatment I dreaded, but the lump got smaller, even though it didn't go completely.

'I thought back over my life. I had never wanted children, but now I felt resentful that I couldn't. For a while I wished I'd had at least one, but in the cold light of day I knew that this was just a panic reaction. Perhaps if the right man had come along, I might have been more maternally minded, but probably not. I wished I'd been closer to my brother and his family; I made up my mind to be a better aunt. I have seen more of them since and am getting to know my niece and nephew.

'Now I feel that I want to be in charge of my life,

however long or short it may be. I want to know what the options are and to feel I am making the choices. I want to retain my dignity and to feel there is an order and reason to what is happening to me. The hysterectomy has paled beside the need for continued treatment of the cancer and I think I may need more. This time I will ask my questions before I agree to any further treatment.'

## LAURA

Laura, married and childless, had a total abdominal hysterectomy with removal of lymph nodes at 24, two years ago. Her ovaries were left. Laura had been married for four years and using the contraceptive pill when she went to the doctor to discuss becoming pregnant.

'The doctor didn't do another cervical smear as it wasn't quite three years since the last one, which had been clear. He said I was in a low-risk category and looked very healthy. Famous last words! A couple of months later I returned after experiencing pain and spotting of blood on intercourse. A relief doctor took a smear and asked about the symptoms. The pain was like someone sticking a knife in me and I thought perhaps it was something silly like thrush, but the doctor asked if I had considered it might be a growth. Three hours later the implications of this hit me. No doctor would worry his patient unless he was positive and I realized that I had something very serious. I tried to prepare my husband, John, without alarming him too much and waited for the result. Some weeks later, the hospital telephoned and asked that I return that afternoon for further tests. I was worried, the NHS does not move with such speed for anything commonplace.

'I had to return for the results, but I just knew it was cancer. I was in a daze, and got through the next week by sheer hard work. I told John I thought it was cancer, but not what I thought the outcome would be. He is not a great one for going into hospitals and very rarely came with me, but he came for the result and waited outside. I wanted it this way and I'm very grateful that the staff always let me do what I wanted, not what they wanted. The consultant said I had a very rare form of cancer of the cervix and that the GP was very good to spot it. I would have to have a radical hysterectomy as soon as possible and a more experienced surgeon at another hospital would do it. I have only praise for the medical teams I have come into contact with, although there were a few misunderstandings and some funny incidents, the care and attention I received was second to none. So I went back to John in the car and told him I had to go in for an operation. We don't talk much about our feelings, we never have, but when we got home I told him it would mean no children. We both had a good cry and then got on with the practical things. We saw the consultant together the next week; I had three weeks before surgery. I was very glad to have this breathing space. It was nice to come to terms with it myself. One of the worst things is to be operated on too quickly, before it has had time to sink in. A lot of women feel cheated out of discussing other possible treatments before the op, not understanding the urgency. I sorted out all the practical details at work and home. I cleaned the house and stocked up the freezer and was very glad I had when I came out.

'I needed someone to talk to, my own doctors were on holiday the week before my operation and I didn't know who else to ask the few questions I had. I felt great shock. I thought a lot about the op, but not too much about its consequences until it was over. One step at a time. I coped so well, because if I had collapsed everyone else around me would too. I felt I was supporting them, instead of it being the other way around. I don't know where I got that strength from. Even after the op, I was told I was too bright and to expect a depression. I'm still waiting! I did not fear cancer or the op itself. I had made up my mind that if I survived the op with no further treatment, all well and good. If I didn't, no problem! I would refuse chemotherapy, as I did not think the treatment justified the ends. This distressed John when I told him after the op and before the results were known.

'John was very upset and worried for me. He found it difficult to accept and to tell other people, and, like me, didn't know how to handle their reactions. I told a close workmate of my husband and he let everyone know at work and arranged compassionate leave for John. John couldn't bring himself to tell our parents either, so I did. It was one of the worst things and there was no easy way, so I just came out with it. John's parents are already grandparents, but John is the only son, so the family name will die with him. Both were concerned, but his father took the news badly and later broke down and cried. My parents are not grandparents, although I have a sister, and they were harder to tell. My father also took it badly, he cried when he came to visit me in hospital. I don't know what it is about fathers.

'I was very anxious in hospital as they didn't give the results of the op until the day of discharge. Another girl of 29, who had the same as me, was told post-op she still had the tumour. I had two days to go and demanded my results, but was told the consultant had not confirmed them yet. I was so annoyed at this reply that even sister couldn't calm me. I was convinced the news was bad or they would have told me. I was told the next morning that everything was perfectly all right, and I still had my ovaries. John's mother was a great help post-op, popping in every day when John returned to work and she did our ironing for three months.

'We told everyone we knew, what op I was having and why. People were upset and concerned. Most said "You'll adopt of course" as if it was a foregone conclusion, which it wasn't. What knocked me for six more than anything else, was what to do for the next twenty to thirty years. I had planned for the next ten years to be taken up with raising a family. Some very good advice was "Don't make any decisions until at least a year post-op'. This would give us time to adjust to the change in circumstances and to learn to live with them. We have gone no further than the reserve waiting list for adoption in our area, having decided for the moment not to adopt. John and I are of the same opinion on this. Now if someone asks why we haven't got any children I say I was ill two years ago and unfortunately can't have them. Most people are satisfied with that. I don't mind too much, but I'm sure other members of the family are upset by the question.

'I feel no different as a woman. My sex life is just as good as before, although I need extra lubrication. I don't feel that anything is missing, except periods and I don't miss those. It seems silly, but I get the urge to wear a bikini now. I've never worn one before as I felt my tummy was too fat and now is no exception, as I've put on a stone in weight! Maybe it's a desire to let people know what I've gone through, as I have a lateral scar from above the belly button to just inside the hairline. The sister on the ward said no one could see I was ill, if I wanted people to know I would have to tell them. It certainly seems easier than trying to hide it. I do feel different, but because of the change of circumstances I've been through, more than anything else. I feel a stronger person and speak my mind more than I used to.

'Unfortunately, I do still get some post-op pain. I had a laparoscopy when adhesions were divided, but it made no difference. Then it was thought to be a trapped nerve for which I've had ultra-sound treatment, in physiotherapy. I was referred to the pain clinic and had steroid injections, which helped, but this hasn't solved the problem. The more I do, the more it hurts. Most days I get on with the pain, but some days it seems a high price to pay for otherwise good health.

'The cancer! My consultant had never seen it before and my doctor did a very good job of spotting it, it's very rare and easily missed. My mother had lost four babies before she fell pregnant with me and was prescribed a hormone to keep the pregnancy. She carried me successfully, but it left me with cancer of the cervix. It is more common in America where the drug was prescribed much more frequently. My mother doesn't know, and I'm not sure how she would cope with the information. My sister knows and has yearly smears, although my mother didn't take the drug while carrying her. My mother-in-law knows, as one of the recognized high-risk factors of cancer of the cervix, is sleeping around. I have been going out with my husband since I was 14, got engaged at 17 and married at 20. I don't care what other people think, and I can't risk that information getting back to my mother. I get on with life, no one knows what is going to happen next and we can't really plan for the future. I don't feel any better for the op as I wasn't ill (luckily) in the first place.'

## KRISTINE

Kristine, a single parent with one teenage child, had a total abdominal hysterectomy at 45, seven years ago. Kristine has a long-term relationship with a married man, separated from his wife.

'I had a positive smear result and went to see the gynaecologist. I had always had heavy bleeds and taking it all together he said a hysterectomy would be a good idea. I didn't know much about hysterectomy, but felt he was giving me good advice, so I agreed.

'My boyfriend moved in with my son while I was in hospital and took time off work when I came home. I didn't discuss the op with him and I wasn't worried about it. I'd been told that thousands of women have this op and it was all very straightforward and quite simple. I didn't think too much about the cancer; after all, it was coming out and there wasn't a panic about it. Apart from terrible wind pains, the post-op time in hospital was quite pleasant. I enjoyed being with the other women and not having to worry about getting to work or running the flat. I went home after ten days.

'Three weeks post-op I began to get pain in my abdominal scar. It had been sore since the op, but became inflamed and angry. A lump developed and then the scar began to ooze, a wound infection! This made me feel very low and took several weeks to clear up with antibiotics and daily dressings. I didn't get any answers to my questions as to why I got an infection and why it took such a long time to clear. It was far more troublesome than the op itself and slowed down my recovery and return to work. I was left with a painful lump on the scar, which took nearly a year to be less sensitive.

'Sex hadn't been a big part of our relationship before the op and I did not intend to resume intercourse afterwards. There was no discussion, I just told my boyfriend it was no longer possible. He could see there were problems with the wound and knew it was very painful for me. He has never pressed the issue and accepts that part of our relationship is over. He was a good help at the time of the op and after. He and my son get along very well, although they are not related.

'Now I am very well and it's hard to remember details. I returned to the hospital a couple of times for high vault smears, but don't go any more. I really don't want to think back too much; I'm very glad to have had the cancer removed completely. It's over and finished with. The hysterectomy wasn't a problem, but I think I should have found out more about it beforehand.'

# 7.
# OVARIAN CYSTS

Ovarian cysts are blister-like formations containing fluid or semi-fluid substances that develop on the ovary. There are several different kinds and a large number, usually growing no bigger than 4 cm, form and disperse over a period of weeks with no treatment. Some occur as part of other conditions, for example, the chocolate cysts of endometriosis, where the blister contains blood. Where the woman is older (40-plus), or the cyst is very large and stuck to the womb, or is part of a large cluster on both ovaries, or is a cancer (often symptomless), hysterectomy is performed with removal of ovary(ies). Symptoms of non-cancerous cysts include pain at site and bleeding irregularities. As there is a chapter on endometriosis, chocolate cysts are not included here.

One of the following four women had an ovarian cancer, one also had fibroids; all are over 35, two are childless.

## MARIA

Maria, single parent of two children, had a total abdominal hysterectomy and remaining ovary removed at 41, seventeen months ago. Maria had already had one ovary removed thirty years ago because of an ovarian cyst.

'At the end of my thirties, my periods got heavier, with huge clots. For over an hour I would have to change a super tampon and giant pad every ten minutes. I would feel dizzy and have to sit down. I had a bloated feeling and some bleeding in the week before my period started. The doctor said it was normal for my age and gave me a smear test! I started getting agonizing pains when my period started and remembered it as the same pain I had when I was a child. I went to Casualty and had a scan but it didn't show anything. I found out afterwards that gas blocks it and I'd drunk fizzy mineral water before the scan. The pain came every other month and when it was bad (worse than labour pains!) I phoned for the ambulance.

'A laparoscopy revealed that my womb and right ovary were enlarged. The houseman gave me some very strong pain-killers and told me there was nothing wrong with me and nothing to worry about! I thought that if there was nothing wrong with me, I wouldn't need pain-killers. The tablets made me extremely sleepy and unable to function normally. The pains continued and I had another scan. This time I drank plain water. My womb was full of fibroids and I had an ovarian cyst, which I could see on the screen as a black hole.

'I was fairly resigned to having a hysterectomy, but I was worried at the prospect of losing my remaining ovary. I had been unable to take the Pill and so was worried about taking hormones. Would I get the right dose? Would I get depressed, grow old, lose my sex drive or grow a beard? I had been sterilized at 28 and had come to terms with not having any more children, so the lack of a womb didn't worry me that way.

'When the doctor, a different one again, told me that I would have to have a hysterectomy, despite expecting it, I broke down in tears. He couldn't cope and so I saw the consultant for the first time. He was very reassuring and positive, but thought the cyst would disintegrate before he operated. I didn't believe him. He would try to save the ovary, but in women over 40, it was considered best to take everything and save trouble later. He wanted to give me a hormone implant, but I wanted to take pills so that I could have some control over the dosage. He tried to talk me out of it, as did another doctor, but I felt strongly about it.

'I was apprehensive during the seven-week wait as I hadn't enjoyed previous operations. The injection in the back of the hand was like dying and I'd had a chest infection once, which was distressing, but the bleeding was a real problem and the pains so bad that I knew it had to be done. I stocked up with lots of food for my daughter (14) and the three cats, and heavy things that I wouldn't be able to carry afterwards.

'In hospital I was so nervous, feeling very alone and frightened and I cried. A couple of nurses came and sat with me; they were very kind and patient, as was the woman doctor. They said it was my body and I didn't have to have the operation, but I knew I did. I felt okay after the pre-med. On the way down to theatre they banged my feet on the wall of the lift, but I was too dozy to do anything about it. I was left with two other women who were upset. They were having abortions and I heard the doctor ask one if she wanted to change her mind. Then they gave me the injection in the back of the hand. It stung.

'When I woke I felt very dopey, and surprised that I didn't feel too much pain. The night nurses were very kind and looked after me. I had a drip and as I couldn't pass water I had a catheter put in next day. I had always dreaded these two things, but the drip was good as I didn't get a terrible thirst and the catheter didn't hurt and meant I could rest. The drip was taken out later and the catheter the next day. I began to feel better, but I had a constant pain at the top of my vagina, and then I was very ill with a temperature. They took a swab from my vagina and a blood test and started me on antibiotics. I couldn't eat at all for one week and the smell of food made me feel sick. When the consultant came round with the entourage, he did an internal. It was very painful and he said "Oh, a haematoma!" I was told to grip the houseman's hand tightly. I was very frightened. The consultant shoved his hand inside me and burst some stitches. It was agony and I screamed. As soon as the blood came down, I felt better and three days later I went home. Being in a twenty-four bedded ward was exhausting as it felt crowded and the others were mostly bladder repairs. Dreadful, a lot worse! I was very tired for a few weeks and slept a lot. Three months later I was feeling better and I started riding and ballet classes again. I still got tired easily and needed lots of sleep.

'I tried making love with a close man friend and felt the usual good feelings, but penetration was agony. I went back to the hospital and was told the scar had overhealed. They painted it with acid a couple of times, but it had no effect. Seven months later, I had an anaesthetic while they burnt the scar tissue away with diathermy. It didn't take long and when I came round it didn't hurt. I had met a wonderful man and two months after the diathermy, when we made love, it didn't hurt!! We will soon be living together and our sex life is fine.

'Looking back, I feel angry that I had to go through so much pain and upheaval before I was finally operated on. I had told them I had an ovarian cyst as it was the same pain as before. I got fed up with seeing a different doctor every time and having to explain everything again and again. It would have been nice to have had a close friend with me before going to theatre, some help with the housework for a couple of weeks post-op, and the diathermy a lot sooner.

'Now seventeen months later, I get an occasional hot flush and my skin is a little drier. I have a problem with weight gain due to the HRT, but I feel very well, very positive and much better than I have for several years. I was worried about depression, but haven't had any. It's wonderful not to menstruate, to always feel okay with no mood swings and not be ruled by my body. I feel much more confident and don't feel any less of a woman. I would recommend the operation for anyone who needs it.

## WINNIE

Winnie, married with two children, 9 and 12 years, had a total abdominal hysterectomy and both ovaries removed four years ago.

'One evening on going to the toilet, I noticed a pain after passing water, but didn't worry unduly. I put it down to something I had eaten, or the fact that my period was due.

My periods were perfectly normal and regular as clockwork. I slept well, but when I woke, the pain was more severe. I experienced difficulty passing water and felt unwell. Although my husband thought I was making a fuss, I went to see the doctor the next day.

'He examined me, gave me some pain tablets, and asked me to return after the weekend for a letter to the hospital. I was very worried, as I guessed he had found something that shouldn't be there. It was three weeks before I saw the gynaecologist and then I felt quite ill, with bad pains in my right shoulder and arm, and down my left side. He said I had a cyst on an ovary that was growing very fast and pushing all my internal organs out of place. He knew I was in great pain and would operate on his next list at that hospital in a fortnight. I was asked if I wanted any more children, but I'd been advised not to. By the time I went into hospital I had a lump sticking out of the bottom of my back and I was told I might have a hysterectomy.

'They took both ovaries out and did a hysterectomy. One ovary had a cyst as big as a grapefruit and the other had several smaller ones. The doctor said: "Well as you didn't want any more children and at your age, we thought it best to take everything." They didn't think the cysts were malignant. It was a small cottage hospital and a local GP called in every morning. He told me not to suffer too much (he didn't say what I might suffer from) and to see my own doctor when I got home. He was very reluctant to discuss anything. I made a reasonable recovery, apart from a wound abscess, but I can't take penicillin so they had to find something else. I went home after fourteen days. I had no one to help me and had been promised a home help. It was a couple of weeks before anyone came and I muddled through with the help of good friends. I was very depressed and low for some time, and had very bad night sweats, which I told the doctor about at my six-week check. He said to try and put up with them as he didn't like giving HRT! He confirmed that the cysts weren't malignant. I asked my own doctor about HRT, but he said

I had to get old and he wouldn't give me anything to stop it. I tried to talk to him several times, but his attitude is that it's over, finished with and that's that!

'I felt a failure. I had both children under anaesthetic and don't know anything about giving birth and I haven't been able to manage the change. Although my friends are now going through the change and I haven't got this to come, I still feel cheated. Several have had a hysterectomy, but have only lost their wombs, and have relief from years of heavy periods. People say: "I expect you wish you'd had this done years ago, you must feel miles better." I was ill for just over four weeks, so while it was a relief from that pain, there was nothing long term I needed relieving.

'I would have liked much more counselling, both before and after. I felt an important part of me had been taken away that would affect my whole life. It seemed as if the doctors thought it was none of my business. I still feel I would like to talk it out with a doctor. Basically I feel you need to take time to recover and then get on with your life. The only help and answers to any of my questions I got from a voluntary group, HSG. Another regret is that now my daughter has started her periods, I'm not as sympathetic as I would have been, if I was still having them. It's surprising how quickly you forget!

'It hasn't made me feel older or worried me that way. Once the first three months were over I have been fine.'

## HEATHER

Heather, married for the second time, had a total abdominal hysterectomy and removal of both ovaries at 45, nine months ago. Heather is childless, all her pregnancies ended in miscarriage. Her husband's daughter from a previous marriage lives with them. Heather is diabetic, asthmatic and has a history of deep-vein thrombosis. On three previous occasions, over nine years, Heather experienced severe pains in her right side. The gynaecologist said there was nothing wrong and diagnosed her as a hypochondriac.

'Eighteen months ago, my periods became very heavy and painful with the gripping pain in the right-hand side. The doctor said it was imaginary, and I carried on. It did no good for my ego to be disbelieved and told that what I felt wasn't there. Then it all felt very wrong and I thought – cancer! The doctor came to my home during a pain attack and found an internal swelling on the right-hand side. A scan showed a cyst on the ovary, but I was told that nothing could be done. I was given pethidine for the pain, but it got worse over the next six months. I saw a gynaecologist who said a hysterectomy and removal of both ovaries should be done. I was worried, but relieved that at last something was being done about it, someone believed me! The anaesthetist discussed the specialist care I would need and said to lose $12\frac{1}{2}$ kg (2 stone) in weight for the operation.

'The pain had stopped my sense of humour and I took it out on my husband and daughter. It affected my marriage and we rowed a lot. My husband would put his arms around me and ask to help, but it hurt my stomach. I pushed him away each time and he felt rejected and thought I had found someone else while he was at work. I built a wall around myself to cope with pain and he couldn't get through. He stopped trying, feeling that I didn't want or love him. When he heard about the hysterectomy, he said: "Thank goodness for that. It's the best thing that could happen." He looked forward to the op, and said it was his fault we had no children.

'A month later I had a cervical smear test and a letter came requesting that I go for a colposcopy. I nearly collapsed, I had an asthma attack. I'd never heard the word before, but felt it meant cancer. The doctor said it was just an abnormal cell structure, but it meant cancer to me! It made me a "high risk" and meant an earlier hysterectomy. The doctor tried to reassure me that the cyst on the ovary was just that, as cancer had a different outline. He reminded me of my medical problems (asthma, etcetera) that get worse when I worry, but I still worried. I did not tell my husband about this, he has had heart problems for four years and needs a beta blocker daily. Stress is bad for him and I felt the less he knew the better. I sat and brooded by myself and things got worse between us. He thought I was going to leave him.

'I found the colposcopy and laser treatment painful. A small wart was also removed and I had an infection for two weeks following this. The next two months until the operation were a nightmare. I lived on my nerves, had tachycardia (palpitations) with anxiety and lots of problems re house and finances. The pethidine didn't work on the pain any more and it was as though I were a zombie. My blood pressure went up and then a cold prevented my admission!

'I was in two minds whether to go ahead and went to see a faith healer. He told me that he couldn't cure me, that I needed surgery and not to delay the operation, as if I did I wouldn't live! Problems came and I cancelled the bed. My GP came to my home and urged me to have it, so I decided I would! Amongst other things, I made a will as it was likely I wouldn't make it with my medical problems. I told my husband about the abnormal cells. He was devastated that I hadn't told him and wanted to know why. He couldn't understand why I bore it alone when we were supposed to be a couple. I couldn't tell him that I'd felt so alone and isolated. I was unsure how he'd take the fact that if I did survive I would have no more reproductive organs. Sex had been a problem for a year, how long before he looked for someone else? There was no way to explain and I just said I was sorry for not telling him and would he bear with me as I was having a trying time.

'I was terrified about the surgery, but the staff were so good, I was quite calm. Apart from saying that they were going to take everything, nothing else was explained. I was very ill afterwards and also had an asthma attack. I had a drip in one hand and a transfusion in the other as well as a drain taking blood and pus off. I felt like hell, but was relieved it was all over. I was told that there hadn't been any sign of cancer and they had taken everything.

'On the fourth day post-op, it suddenly hit me that I was no longer what I would class as a true female. I cried and dripped in sorrow for myself. One nurse was so shocked, she didn't know what to say. The other nurse lived two streets away from me and was quite different. "Instead of sitting there in self pity, you should thank God your life was saved. That wasn't just a cyst on your ovary, there was an abscess spilling out pus. Another forty-eight hours and you would've been dead!" I did thank God.

'I went home after two weeks with lots of antibiotics. I was in pain, but calm. The discharge got worse, as did the pain and discomfort. I was used to being active, but spent eight weeks in a wheelchair, unable to bend or stand. I had a home help and meals on wheels and spent my time sleeping and going to the loo and bathroom to change towels. I felt much worse than I did pre-op. During this time I had big rows with my husband.

'On my return to hospital, the doctors were shocked at the discharge and stench, which was due to a bad pelvic infection. Trying to fight this off was bad enough as a diabetic, but then I was hit by menopausal symptoms, and had trouble with the deep veins in my legs. The doctor gave me more antibiotics and pain-killers. I couldn't have HRT, not sure that I would've taken it anyway. It was a terrible time. I experienced spells of amnesia at home and worried that I might end up shoplifting, so I didn't go shopping on my own for a while. I now have a mild tranquillizer and antidepressant. I thought at one stage I was going mad and feared being put in a mental hospital. I eventually found help by contacting Claire of the HSG. She was my saviour by explaining about the menopause and just being there at the other end of the phone.

'Five months later I was gradually getting better and people were saying: "You've had a hysterectomy, you must feel like a new woman." I looked for the nearest object to hit them with! Suddenly I was ill again. A stomach bug followed by flu, followed by a middle ear infection that caused me to vomit every time I moved my head. The pain was treated with pethidine again. It was my lowest ebb and I cried all day in self-pity. I cried for the babies I'd lost, the children I'd never had. I cried because I'd been adopted and no one has ever belonged to me. I felt old, I looked old; I thought, I'm no longer a woman!

'In the evening, I sat down to work my life out. I couldn't think my way out of the menopause, it was real, but my body was not going to rule me. There are alternatives to HRT on the homeopathic side. So I saw a homeopathist. The bad flushes were helped by salvia and sepia works for other menopausal symptoms. My dry skin was helped by a Vit E cream and I experimented with different shades of make-up. I changed my hair colour.

'My attitude! Looking on the dark side of things was seriously affecting my life, so I tried to have a happy outlook. If I was down or depressed I would sing or dance to a record. I am a completely different character now in hair, make-up, and clothes, as if to substitute for not being a true female. Oh, I know I am a female, but not a reproducing one. I work that little bit harder to keep my husband's interest in me and stop him looking outside the home.

'After the ear infection I had another pelvic infection. This cleared up with a course of antibiotics from the GP. I had also lost my job through so much illness. This had been important to me not just for financial reasons.

'My husband and I eventually sat and talked everything through. He had felt panic-stricken and unable to cope with all that was going on. We have a better understanding of each other now and have stopped leading separate lives of misery. He is just glad that I made it and the reproductive organs bit doesn't matter at all to him. He sees me as a complete female and doesn't know what he'd do without me. It was the best thing to do and I wish I had done it before. We're both relieved it's over and that I'm clear of cancer. It is perhaps harder on the man, as there is no way to explain what a woman goes through. It is easier for her to curl up in a ball and live in her world of misery, one a man can't get into.

'Sex was difficult afterwards, I was afraid of the pain

and he was afraid of hurting me. After a couple of failures I felt he didn't want me. Then when we got that sorted out and had sex it did hurt, but I didn't let it show. I realized that I had another pelvic infection. I hope it will be better for me soon. I wish I'd known that being diabetic made me susceptible to a pelvic infection post-op and to infections like flu during the first year.

'I am still very angry with the gynaecologist who originally said there was nothing wrong. I cannot forgive him. Marriage and children go together and most women, unless they don't want children, assume that they will have children. I was adopted and I badly needed someone of my own, someone who was a part of me, who was from me. It hurts and hurts very deeply that I haven't had that child because of a gynaecologist who dismissed me as a hypochondriac.'

## SALLY

Sally, divorced and childless, had a total abdominal hysterectomy with removal of both ovaries at 37, ten months ago. Her ex-husband had been promiscuous and knowing this Sally's doctor had sent for her, eleven months ago, to have a cervical smear. Sally's last smear, a year before, had been clear.

'I read the letter and wept, with shock, with anger at my ex-husband, and fright. Had he given me AIDS and was this a tactical way to call me in? I went a few weeks later, irritated at the inconvenience. I had experienced some discomfort, was tender and hurt on examination. My tummy was enlarged and I had a lot of flatulence. The doctor did a pregnancy test, amusement lightened the tension, was this a late pregnancy? Excitement! I imagined holding and caring for a baby. What sex would it be? Anxiety! I was alone in a small, gardenless cottage, in the centre of town. Not suitable. The result was negative. Disappointment and relief, and the doctor referred me to the gynaecology clinic. I was shaken by the speed, the appointment was the next week. I went, irritated at the inconvenience and another internal examination, but happy and relaxed. The doctor examining me asked how soon I could go in. I said "I'm here". A silly thing to say! I had "something" on my ovaries and was to be admitted in two days time! Shock. Terror. Numb disbelief and alarm bells.

'I rang around and made arrangements; I would take my cats, "my babies", down to my parents. I prepared for the worst, but hoped it would be all right. Everyone I spoke to had been sympathetic, concerned, with lots of offers of help. I kept busy, but was in a dream, nothing seemed real. I couldn't believe it, this happened to other people. Driving to deliver the cats I had time for reflection. No one had mentioned hysterectomy and it wasn't a serious consideration. We are not a communicative family, but my father was more supportive than my mother. Although she'd had a hysterectomy, it was all a little "dirty", certainly embarrassing and she didn't want to talk.

'Gerald, a recent, past boyfriend, heard the news and insisted on taking me to hospital. I don't know who was most nervous. I was anxious and aware of the implications, but shied away from thinking about them. It was a bit of an adventure, I'd be out in a few days! The tests were to take several days, so bang went that hope. The scan was during lunch. Don't hospitals have a talent for ruining meals one way or another? In fact it was my one and only test!

'Hysterectomy was mentioned. HORROR. PANIC. TERROR. DESPAIR. Later, ANGER. I needed more time, I hadn't used my bits yet. How pathetic we must seem as we try to alter the wording on the consent form and need persuading that hysterectomy is only done as a life-saving measure. My feelings fluctuated all day. Visitors saved my sanity – my closest friends – and they were *there*, sympathetic and concerned. I had butterflies getting ready for theatre.

'Post-op, I was overwhelmed with pain. Morphia helped me through, but I was hardly lucid for three days. I was

devastated and totally lethargic and disinterested in the
world outside, and my cats! I clung to the past and
hankered after the time when I was still whole, the ostrich
syndrome! So much despair, anger and tears. Too late.
Too late. Too late. Despair, anger and tears, a vicious
circle. I went to my parents at the end of the week.

'I was looked after wonderfully well, but not allowed to
talk about it, which I needed to do. I tried and was told
very abrasively by my mother that it was too late anyway!
I was so full of despair and as I got stronger, regret became
apparent and has never disappeared. Anger was too tiring
and I needed strength. I wept in bed every morning, it
would not have been tolerated otherwise. My mother
couldn't understand what was so upsetting, she'd been
glad to get rid of hers! Friends were marvellous and
telephoned every day.

'It had been cancerous and I needed chemotherapy. I
felt relieved to be coming home. Despair and regret, now
rage returned. Friends from years ago started crawling out
of the woodwork as word got round. At last I could talk,
and talk I did, and raged at the injustice of it all. I still
cried in the mornings, but would erupt at any time. I had a
Macmillan cancer nurse, who realized that the
hysterectomy troubled me more than the cancer and so
that's what we talked about. She also arranged a home
help.

'I felt physically empty and that my stomach would
drop out if I moved suddenly and bad, hot flushes started
a week post-op. After eight weeks the GP gave in and gave
me HRT pills. What bliss. Now I felt like a teddy bear
with no stuffing! My parents still worried about the
cancer, of which I'd been cleared, and telephoned more
often to talk about this, but never the op. Friends have
been marvellous in all ways, loads of moral support and
listening time! I was lucky to have a woman doctor, who
spent many hours sitting and talking to me, with diagrams
etcetera. She was just as concerned with my mental
wellbeing.

'I have had difficulty coming to terms with the

hysterectomy, after all I will get over the cancer, but will never recover my uterus. A ship without a sail. The difficulty is intensified by the fact I haven't any children. I felt isolated although I knew differently. This year has gone frighteningly quickly. My anger has gone completely. Despair never will and sometimes overwhelms me. I know I have friends of the best quality and that helps. If I had my time over again, I'd be a teenage mum!'

# 8.
# PELVIC INFLAMMATORY DISEASE (PID)

PID is infection in the pelvic area, most commonly in the Fallopian tubes; it can spread to the ovaries and surrounding tissue, flaring up at intermittent intervals. Often the symptoms, low pelvic pain, bloated stomach, irregular bleeding, vaginal discharge, plus general flu-like symptoms, are not recognized by the woman and it may be some years before a diagnosis is made. By this time the PID is chronic and has probably caused scarring with adhesions sticking the ovaries and tubes to the womb and other pelvic organs. PID can occur after any pelvic surgery, for example, appendicitis, abortion, D and C, sterilization, hysterectomy, after childbirth or as a result of sexually transmitted disease. The ages of the four women in this chapter range from 22 to 35. All have children. For two, PID occurred after having a baby; for another, symptoms became apparent after an emergency appendicectomy. One also had her ovaries and tubes removed.

## LISA

Lisa, married with one child, had a total abdominal hysterectomy at 32, four years ago.

'My problem started after I had my first and only child. I began to get severe shooting pains in my vagina and up into my stomach. It was like somebody sticking sharp swords up my vagina when I was walking, sitting or lying down. I was referred by my family doctor to a (woman)

gynaecologist and was under her for three years before I
had a laparoscopy. I was told I had an infection in the
tubes and a few months later had twelve weeks of deep
heat treatment. They had said it wasn't 100 per cent
certain whether the pain would clear up and it didn't.
In the end they told me I was imagining the pain.

'I went back to my doctor and asked for a second
opinion. He referred me to another hospital and a (male)
gynaecologist. I was given four months treatment of
tablets and pessaries for the pain and infection. The pain
continued and on my son's fifth birthday, I was told I had
PID and only a hysterectomy would help. I had had pain
for five years and I was so relieved, for at long last
someone had listened to what was wrong with me. I
jumped off the couch and gave the doctor a kiss. The
operation was booked for two months time.

'My husband, Dan, was very worried about the pains I
was getting and was pleased something was going to be
done. We knew nothing about hysterectomy and weren't
given any information at all. There was nothing in the
library and it was difficult to find out anything. Nobody
wanted to talk about what was going on and really I didn't
have a clue. I heard Sally Haslett (Hysterectomy
Counsellor) on Capital Radio and rang in to her. She was
very helpful and suggested I buy a book from Smith's, but
they didn't have it. Dan thought there should be some
meetings along the lines of ante-natal care, like when we
had our baby, but there was nothing. He wanted to do
what was best for me and felt strongly that I needed his
support, but didn't know exactly how to go about it. My
mum was a little shocked, because it hadn't happened in
the family before. The only thing I was worried about was
that I wouldn't come round from the anaesthetic.

'After the operation I was a few days coming round, but
I did. They had taken everything except my ovaries. I had
a blood-stained discharge for six weeks, with a recurrence
of pain and had a few ups and downs. The doctor said
these were due to my body getting back to normal. I was
left with a feeling of numbness over my scar, which lasted

about a year and then wore off. Dan was very supportive before and after the operation, helping me in all different ways. We went to some HSG meetings which helped us both, as we found out a lot that we wanted to know and it helped to see how different people coped.

'We had hoped to have another baby, but nothing happened, so it hurt me at first. It was very hard to realize, even afterwards, I couldn't have any more. Sometimes I felt down, especially one time when my friends all had babies. It was hard to get over, but I did. I came to the conclusion that it's the best thing I could've had done.

'I had another attack of pain about eighteen months afterwards and I went immediately to the doctor. It cleared very quickly with a course of antibiotics and I've not had any more.

'Sex has stopped altogether, but that is due to me and not the operation. I just don't have any feelings about wanting it. I did go for counselling about this, but all the doctor did was listen to me and so I stopped going. My husband also has been seriously ill for a couple of years now with bad heart trouble and needs heart surgery.

'Sometimes I wonder, but when I think of all the pain I was in, I know I did the right thing. I am slimmer and my shape has come back, my high stomach has gone down. I work full time, do keepfit and swimming for exercise, and I can sit in chairs and do many things I couldn't do for over five years. I feel I should've had it years sooner.'

## DIANE

Diane, married with a family, had a total abdominal hysterectomy at 35, eleven months ago.

'I suffered a great deal of pain and discomfort with PID for three years. During my illness I felt I was pushed from pillar to post by the medical profession, at a time when I was least able to help myself. After two years of trying this treatment and that – antibiotics, diathermy, for instance – I was put on the list for a hysterectomy. Nothing was explained to me, except that I had not responded to treatment. I was told that I was lucky that I could have the inflamed area removed, unlike a bronchial sufferer. I did not feel "lucky" and told my doctor so. He asked if I wanted any more children and when I said no, his reply was: "What use is your womb then? You don't need it any more!"

'The pain got worse during the year I waited for the hysterectomy. I was not told what to expect afterwards and received no information whatsoever. On the night before my op my husband was asked to go into the sister's office alone, while I stood outside. *He* had to sign forms agreeing that he was aware *he* could not have children any more. I think there is a total lack of understanding by the medical profession with regard to how a woman feels about hysterectomy. They left my ovaries.

'Since the hysterectomy, I have suffered urinary problems, thrush, hormonal imbalance and depression. I had taken hormones for a hormone imbalance pre-op, but was told to stop taking these after the op. All my symptoms of painful breasts and PMT have recurred. I had no counselling and felt distraught, but the hospital discharged me, even though I told them how unwell I was. I was advised to take up a hobby and forget my symptoms!

'The usual comment by people on hearing I'd had a hysterectomy was that it would make me a new woman. It did. Around two months post-op, I hardly recognized myself. I was tired, depressed and very emotional. I went from tears to screaming in minutes. I felt unattractive and self-conscious about the scar on my tummy and couldn't understand why my husband still fancied me. He was very patient, doing his best to assure me that he loved me.

'I started antidepressants and a nurse called weekly to teach me relaxation. The PMT became very severe and for two weeks each month I was an argumentative, raving lunatic. Then recently, my doctor prescribed me the hormone progesterone. It seems to be my life-saver, but why, oh why, was it refused post-op? It could have saved

my family and myself a year of suffering. Antidepressants were handed out too easily, treating the
symptoms rather than the cause. I am still suffering from
thrush and cystitis, to which no amount of hobbies make a
difference.

'Since starting the progesterone, I'm beginning to see
the light at the end of the tunnel. I am feeling much better,
calmer and more able to cope.'

## REBECCA

Rebecca, in a stable relationship with two children from
her first marriage, had a total abdominal hysterectomy at
34, nine months ago. Rebecca first experienced symptoms
the year following her first baby, fourteen years ago, but
wasn't diagnosed as PID until recently.

'I got no joy from my doctor, and I just soldiered on,
making the best of the good days! It was like having a
nagging toothache but there were times when all seemed to
be well. Six years ago I had a really severe attack again,
backache and pain, with periods every fortnight. The
doctor tried hormones and this didn't work. After
numerous examinations and smear tests, I was told there
was nothing wrong with me, and if there was, I would just
have to live with it! I felt so ill, I really wondered if I had
lost my sanity. I should have gone for a second opinion,
but I felt that as he was the doctor, he knew what he was
talking about. I plodded on in spite of being absolutely
devastated some days.

'A year ago having separated from my husband and
living with someone else, I put the exhaustion and
frequent periods down to the stress of the marriage break-
up. Then I had difficulty passing water, a problem related
to PID and my new doctor gave me antibiotics for a
bladder infection. When weeks later things were still the
same, the usual routine of tests and examinations began. I
lost count of the internal examinations I had! All came up
with absolutely nothing. Then my partner suggested I see
a gynaecologist who his ex-wife, Gill, had seen four years

earlier. It would mean going privately, but the money for the consultation would be well worth it.

'After an eternity of trying to find out what was really wrong, the gynaecologist told me I had PID and had been suffering with it since the birth of my daughter. Everything fell into place like the pieces of a jigsaw. I shall never forget the wonderful feeling of relief when I was told. I wasn't glad I was ill, but at least I knew what I was dealing with. The consultant was a rarity, someone who explained everything to me. I found that most doctors are too busy to explain anything. He recommended a course of short-wave diathermy to begin with, but if it didn't work felt that hysterectomy was the only option. This was rather a shock, but he was very reassuring and said it would be a last resort, as though fairly common, it was still major surgery. The treatment was quite painless, but everything seemed to get worse even after treatment had stopped. Everything seemed blurred by the absolutely awful pain and the doctor said the only option left was hysterectomy.

'I had never felt so alone and was aware that in the end I had to face this ordeal on my own. I didn't want any more children and my partner had had a vasectomy, so it wasn't difficult in that sense. It was accepting the fact that I was going to lose something of myself. It had caused me so much trouble, but it had always been there, making its presence felt every month. I remember weeping when I had my very last period, it was as though I was grieving for a friend I was about to lose. I found Gill greatly supportive and talked my feelings through with her. I asked her so many things (she had had a hysterectomy) that I was prepared for what was going to happen. I got a helpful book and felt a little knowledge took a great deal of fear out of the situation. It also helped me to ask more constructive questions of the doctors and nurses.

'The consultant I had seen did the op on the NHS. The staff were very helpful and they seemed to care for me as a person, rather than as a body with something wrong with it. I found all this very reassuring as over the years I had lost faith in the medical profession. The ten days in hospital, despite the pain, were not as bad as I had feared.

'Returning home I was shocked by how little I could do. I found getting out of bed and having a bath tired me beyond belief. An independent person by nature, I found depending on others very difficult. I felt I'd not only lost part of myself on a physical level, but in other ways I wasn't the same person. I was dreadfully weepy and would cry for no reason at all. I burst into tears when a friend sent me some flowers to welcome me home!

'When I first went out on my own, I looked around, wondering how many other women in the street had lost their wombs. In that moment I felt very isolated and different. I did worry at one stage that I was less feminine and at that time I did feel less attractive. I had caught a glimpse of myself in the mirror and looked at this body which was far different to before the op, with the scar and a stomach that looked four months pregnant. Now as time passes I feel more in harmony with my body than before and there is a greater freedom sexually.

'Pre-op, I dreaded intercourse because of the pain, then post-op I seemed to have no sexual desire at all. It was as though everything had just been switched off. I worried if orgasm would be the same, and whether I would feel a desire for sex at all. I am pleased to say the desire returned after we made love for the first time. Maybe it was just the fear of nothing being the same that blocked the feeling. Pre-op I used to dry up completely during intercourse, adding to the pain. This has improved markedly and the sexual experience is more intense now. Through all this, my partner has been very understanding and sympathetic and didn't push me into resuming our sexual relationship. I think if I had been pressured, it would have made the fears even greater. He has always treated me as the same person I was before the op. He is relieved for the most part that I am relatively pain free.

'It was a shock that PID could recur after hysterectomy, which can alleviate rather than cure PID. I had thought the op would end all the problems. I suffered an attack three months post-op; nothing like as severe as previously and for which I had antibiotics. I am still finding tiredness a problem and have stiffness and some backache.

'My main feeling about the whole experience was how little I knew about what was happening to me. There seems to be so little written about hysterectomy and PID. I'd never heard about PID until this last year, and I found the information I needed years too late. How frightening it is to realize there are times when doctors can't tell you what's wrong. How many other women are walking around thinking they are imagining their symptoms? Maybe I'm bitter in this respect, but because of the ineptitude of some doctors, I'm left with a condition which will always overshadow my life and with the knowledge of hindsight, it seems so unnecessary.

'Hysterectomy is surrounded by many myths. Some of my friends seemed to think that my life would never be the same again and others, more positively, said it would make a "new woman" of me. I must say that I've found the actual experience to be somewhere between the two. I don't feel any regret about the operation because I have been relieved from suffering a pain to which there seemed to be no end.'

## ALESHA

Alesha, a single parent with one child, had a total hysterectomy and both ovaries removed at 22, three years ago. Alesha's grandparents came to England over forty years ago from Jamaica. Both Alesha and her mother were born in England.

'My problems started after I had an emergency appendicectomy when I was 14. I began to get very heavy periods with pain on the right side. I was told that I would grow out of this, but it got worse as I got older. They were really bad cramping pains and the bleeding would sometimes be every other week. It made me very miserable, tired and irritable, but I didn't like going to the

doctor's much. I set up with my boyfriend when I was
17 and after a few months he made me see my doctor.
I was told it would all clear up after I had a baby. It all
got much worse after I had my baby, eighteen months
later.

'Sex could be really bad at times and at others no
problem, but the good times were getting less. I had loads
of rows with my boyfriend and we broke up a couple of
times. I collapsed a couple of times and eventually my
boyfriend took me to his doctor. He said I had PID, a very
bad infection in my womb and tubes, and gave me stronger
pain-killers and some antibiotics. I had to rest for two
weeks and then see the doctor again. I didn't go back.

'Those last few years were a bad time with the pain,
bleeding and trying to look after my daughter. My mum
was really good and did a lot for me that way. Then I
collapsed with a big bleed and terrible pain and ended up
in hospital. I was there a week, having blood and stuff, and
I saw a gynaecologist who advised a hysterectomy. I really
didn't want to mess about any more and agreed. I had it
two months later; I was 22.

'After the op, they told me they'd taken my ovaries as
well, as I'd been one big mess of adhesions, pus, and
infection inside. They said I was lucky to have had a baby
at all as the tubes, especially the right one, were so twisted
and stuck, and had been for years. I was ill afterwards and
needed a lot of help. My mum helped out mostly, my
boyfriend had gone and at that stage I really didn't care. I
suppose at the time I didn't think much about having the
hysterectomy or having any more children, and it hasn't
bothered me since.

'I was given an implant of hormones (HRT) and this
has been a problem. Each implant leaves a little white scar
on my black skin and it's really ugly. I've had quite a few
now and they look like chickenpox scars on my belly and
thighs. The op scar isn't too bad at all, but these other
scars I don't like. I tried pills for a while, but these didn't
suit me. I tried not having anything and it was hell!

'Sex is okay, no more bad pain; I get a few aches on the

right hand side every now and again. I've had boyfriends since, who've been very macho, wanting a baby as a badge of manhood or virility. Tough! That's their problem; it's not mine and they haven't bothered me. One boyfriend said he would only stay if I had a baby; I can do without that. I don't tell them I've had the op.

'I was so ill, I was just a rag. I couldn't enjoy much or look forward to anything. I think the hysterectomy saved my life and I've done a lot more since I had it. I'm now at college and looking forward to having a career and hardly think about it. Maybe I'll feel bad about it when I'm old, but not now.'

# 9.
# EMERGENCY HYSTERECTOMY

There are so many occasions when life doesn't go as planned and emergency operations are necessary because life is threatened by the unexpected. It is shocking that things have gone wrong, completely shattering and mind-blowing if hysterectomy is the only answer when you are young. All gynaecological surgery carries a risk, and even the simplest like a D and C can go sadly wrong if the womb is punctured. An 18-year-old to whom this happened came round from the anaesthetic to find that a hysterectomy had been done as the only way to stop the bleeding. A similar risk lies in sterilization and one lady, dreadfully upset to find she'd had to have an emergency hysterectomy, was plunged even further into depression by the comment that it could hardly matter to her as she didn't want babies anyway, hence the sterilization!

Sometimes it seems that nature plays a most cruel trick and the longed-for pregnancy takes place, but in the Fallopian tube, where it ruptures. Hysterectomy can save the mother's life but at a cost she may find hard to bear, such as when the rupture of a previous Caesarian Section scar in pregnancy results in hysterectomy, saving the mother's life, but not the baby's. Sometimes, we choose to delay a planned hysterectomy for good reasons, or simply because we just don't recognize the danger signals. Sometimes we hope to get away without actually having one, but it doesn't always work. Fibroids can degenerate, ovarian cysts can undergo torsion (twisting) and of course life can at any time throw up the unexpected, making the hysterectomy an emergency measure.

The four women who had emergency hysterectomies in

this chapter are aged between 25 and 62; three have children, one is childless.

## RUTH

Ruth, married with one child, had an emergency total abdominal hysterectomy at 25, following delivery of her first baby, five years ago. Ruth had become pregnant with the contraceptive coil still in place, but she and her husband, James, were delighted, even though the pregnancy was unplanned. They had been reassured that the coil would not harm the baby. The pregnancy went well but labour was long and unproductive and forceps were applied, unsuccessfully. An emergency Caesarian Section (LSCS) was performed and Ruth had a live baby boy, Simon. Post-op, Ruth was discharged home on the tenth day, breast-feeding the baby. Her husband, a policeman, had six days at home before returning to work on an early shift.

'About mid-day, fifteen days post-birth, I fed Simon on one breast and went to change his nappy. As I did so, I felt a sudden "gush" on my sanitary towel and then liquid was running down my legs. I looked and saw I was covered in bright red blood and then more gushed down my legs. I grabbed a handful of toilet roll, but it was soon soaked in blood. I rushed down the stairs and the blood dripped on the carpet and splashed the bannisters. I was wearing a pair of sandals and the feet indentations were full of blood. I didn't know what to do. I telephoned my neighbour who came, sent me to bed and phoned for the doctor. I was now passing blood clots. The doctor said I had had a post-partum haemorrhage, explaining that if a small part of the placenta was left in the womb, fourteen days later this would cause a haemorrhage. I had been told that the placenta was complete. He sent for an ambulance. I passed out and came to in the ambulance, with an oxygen mask over my face and my feet raised. My son was taken with me.

'I was told off by the admissions sister for not bringing

my co-operation card with me! The ambulance man pointed out that I was in no fit state to bring anything. I was put to bed without pillows and the foot of the bed was raised. I was examined by three doctors and one doctor sat me up, but as I began to faint, he laid me down. I was again given oxygen and the foot of the bed was raised even higher. I had an internal examination and clots of blood were removed. I was given an injection of Ergometrine and a drip containing Syntocinon was put in my arm to control the bleeding. I was given three units of blood and had a D and C and was sent home two days later. I asked if any of the placenta had been found, but the nurses didn't know.

'On day twenty-two post-baby, alone in the evening, I had fed Simon and was changing his nappy. I felt a "gush" on my sanitary pad, and the blood ran down my legs, seeping through my skirt. It was happening all over again! I went to bed, my neighbour called the doctor. I was very frightened and panicky, I felt I couldn't take any more. The doctor was very embarrassed. I had got pregnant on the coil, had an emergency LSCS after a failed forceps delivery, and now a second haemorrhage! I was crying and very upset. I again passed out going to the ambulance. I had the same treatment in hospital as before with several internal examinations. They wanted to know how much blood I had lost but I just didn't know. I had a drip in one arm and blood going into the other; the foot of the bed was raised. I was very uncomfortable and my arms ached. My breasts filled with milk and became engorged, a nurse expressed this for me. I felt extremely depressed and low and cried. I was discharged three days later.

'The next day I had my *third* haemorrhage, I knew exactly what was happening and called my husband. We asked the doctor when he came why it kept happening. He said that if we didn't get a satisfactory answer from the hospital this time, he would find out for us. Again I had the same treatment: Ergometrine, Syntocinon and was examined by several doctors. I felt extremely low and depressed. Next day I was sat out of bed in a chair when I felt the familiar "gush" and there was blood running down my legs, seeping through my nightdress. I couldn't move, either to reach the emergency bell, or the bed. A domestic help came by and got the nursing staff. I had drips put into both arms, which were very sore; my veins kept "blocking up", and the drips weren't working well. I was very upset. "Never mind, at least we can really see what has been happening, I'm not saying we didn't believe you before," said the nurse! By now I feared for my life, I felt so low.

'My consultant, with a lot of other doctors, came to see me that afternoon, the first time since I'd had the baby. I asked her what would happen if the bleeding didn't stop. She was hopeful it would, if it didn't she'd have to take my womb away. I was devastated, I couldn't believe what she had said. Before I could ask any more she had left the room. A haematologist came later and checked my blood-clotting abilities. He didn't think I had a blood disorder, but had been asked to make sure. After the tests he said everything was basically normal, though slow due to my present condition.

'I was crying frequently and becoming more depressed. I was unable to feed my baby many times and my milk was expressed for him. On one occasion the milk was sent to the special-care baby unit and he was fed on bottle milk! Problems with the drips in my arms continued and I spent a very disturbed night. The next day the consultant came and examined me and I felt she had started another haemorrhage. She looked at the pad and said I was just passing stale blood and left the nurses to blanket bathe me. I bled heavily and eventually the consultant was recalled. This was the *fifth* haemorrhage.

'I was told that my womb would have to be removed and that it would be done that afternoon. I was very upset. I didn't want a hysterectomy because I wanted more children and I was only 25 years old. I cried non-stop as the nurses prepared me for the operation. The room seemed full of people and I could hear my baby crying in his cot in the corner of the room. No one seemed to be taking any notice of him and I screamed at them to see to him. A nurse was told to see to him and I was told to calm down. My husband arrived for visiting, but I couldn't stop crying. I was very frightened. I signed the consent form for hysterectomy and was told that I wouldn't be able to have any more babies. They had trouble putting up another drip and the anaesthetist arrived to ask me lots of questions. The room seemed full of people and I couldn't believe this was happening to me. I felt so confused and frightened. I said goodbye to my husband outside the operating theatre and I wondered if I would come out alive. I was very upset and the nurse kept telling me to calm down.

'When I came round, my stomach hurt and I was shaking. I couldn't make out if I was cold or just shaking. I drifted in and out of sleep, and have memories of my husband being there, the nurses taking my pulse, and feeling very thirsty. I felt very weak and couldn't believe what had happened to me. I gave up breast-feeding.

'I was in hospital for another week. I asked the consultant why I had to have the op and was told that a stitch had come out in my womb from the LSCS. She sounded almost embarrassed. I asked if anything else could go wrong and was told that I'd had my fair share of the NHS. I was stunned and didn't know what to say. Later I was sitting in the garden outside the ward, with quiet tears rolling down my face. I felt so very lonely, I was the only young woman there. A female doctor a few years older than myself asked why I was crying. When told that I hurt, she said there was no need, I could have pain-killers. I told her it wasn't physical pain, but emotional pain and that I didn't know how to cope with it. I felt very panicky with it, so much so, I wanted to scream. (I had this feeling many times over the next few years.) The doctor put it down to post-baby blues and couldn't understand what I meant. It had nothing to do with the baby. The word HYSTERECTOMY was constantly running through my mind in big, bold letters as if on a ticker-tape machine. I was 25, I felt that I should be looking forward to my life, but something had died within me. It was as if my life was on the decline and I was getting ready to die, as an old person would slow down and lose their faculties. It frightened me, I was losing twenty years of my life, facing a situation that many women face when 45 years old and going through the menopause.

'At the post-op check I was sent in to see the family planning officer who asked about my blood loss! I had to explain I'd had a hysterectomy and became very distressed. My consultant made a joke about hay fever when she came into the room! I was never given any real help by hospital or GP. I felt I was passed from one to the other, always being told I would get over it. Perhaps I would, but how did I cope with the feelings of desperation at that time? I attempted to get help for my emotional needs, but was told to pull myself together as there was no one to help me. Had I got a church minister to see? All the time they insisted that it was post-natal depression. I felt like screaming: "It is POST-HYSTERECTOMY DEPRESSION and that is something quite different!"

'When I met other mums at the baby clinic, the subject soon came around to labour, contraception, and planning the next baby. All I can say is, How I hated those women! They had something that I didn't have, the ability to have children, the need for contraception and yes, that badge of a woman, a monthly period. I was so jealous I felt almost violent towards them. (I've never shared these feelings before as I've been so ashamed of how I felt.) I frowned a lot in those days. I was really worried that if I felt like this when I had a baby, how would I feel when I hadn't and desperately wanted another one? We were told we could adopt, but I was adamant that I wanted my own baby or none at all. I had fantasies of becoming pregnant, a miracle mum with an artificial womb or transplant. I even wrote to a famous obstetrician. When friends became pregnant, I became totally oblivious to them. I never asked how they were, did my best to avoid contact and worst, ignored them. My husband asked me if I wanted to lose all my friends, as my attitude was leading to just that. I was

desperately jealous and hoped that something would go
wrong for them as it had for me!

'I've never felt close to my mother, and she's never
asked or shown any interest in how I felt about the
hysterectomy. My sister, (with three children!) told me
bluntly that I should be thankful I have one child and am
alive. My brother, four years older than me, probably
doesn't even know what happened to me. My older
brother, to whom I was very close, is a Methodist minister.
He had been married fourteen years when I had my
hysterectomy and thought that he and his wife couldn't
have children. Within a year they had a son, followed two
years later by a girl. I felt that I had to lose my womb for
them to have children. I was very close to him and so was
very upset when he felt unable to tell me that they were
expecting their second baby. I've hardly spoken to him
since and have never seen the baby. I tried to make up,
but his wife didn't want to see me. When my other
brother's daughter was christened I was asked not to
go so that I wouldn't upset my elder brother's wife!
My husband's family have never said very much
apart from a memorable quote from Grandma: "If I
can get over it at 81, I'm sure that Ruth will be able to
at 25!"

'My husband and I had been a happy, young, married
couple, sex was a pleasure in itself. Post-op I almost hated
him when my depression was bad and felt that he didn't
care what happened to me. He wanted life to continue as
normal, something I couldn't do. I was very cold towards
him, common courtesy and affection were minimal and
sex non-existent. My views had changed. Sex had one
purpose: to have babies. Since I couldn't have babies, why
bother? Things came to a head when I realized suddenly
what I was doing and wondered how he had stood me like
that for over a year. I promised myself I would make an
effort to become "normal" again. It has been slow and I've
slid back down the road to depression many times. During
those first eighteen months I thought seriously about
suicide. Why didn't I do it? I did want all the pain, anger,

hurt, bitterness and depression to go away, but I didn't want to die.

'Now, five years later, life is . . . well, LIFE IS!! Our sex life is normal. I know that my vagina is closed and I feel sad that I can never take my husband's semen deep within me. I feel a little "cut off" and of course we'll never have that accident that makes us OAP parents! The anger at the hospital staff will never, never, never go away. Whether it was medical fluke or their fault that I needed the op, they treated me awfully.

'I will never get over having a hysterectomy. Recently a friend had the same experience. I had been close to her during the pregnancy and helped care for her toddler. When I heard what had happened, every bitter, hurt, angry, frightening memory came back. Also I felt that in some way I was responsible for what had happened to her. Perhaps if I hadn't been her friend, it wouldn't have happened! Stupid isn't it? No, I won't get over the hysterectomy, *but* I have learned to live and cope with the outcome of it. It has robbed me of an awful lot of things, *but* it has also made me richer in other ways. We have adopted a baby boy, a brother for Simon, and he has made us a proper family. I have a husband who has stood by me; I know what real pain is and feel that I am, consequently, a wiser person.'

## PAT

Pat Reid came to England from Jamaica in 1962 and has worked as a health professional ever since. Pat, married with two children, was 42 when she had an emergency total abdominal hysterectomy four years ago.

'When my first baby was born, fifteen years ago, the midwife thought I had twins because I also had large fibroids. The consultant said I would have to have them out at a later date if they didn't go down after the birth. I was much more worried that, when ten weeks' pregnant, I had suffered a deep vein thrombosis (DVT) and spent five weeks in hospital with a pulmonary embolism. This meant that whenever I had to have an operation, or treatment of any kind, I would have to mention this and the fact that I had had the drug Warfarin prophylacticly (as a preventative measure). The fibroids did go down, but raised their ugly heads again when I was carrying my second child, two years later. I was advised not to have any more children after this one.

'My periods were very heavy with clots, and lasted seven to nine days; I needed two or three pads at a time. I suffered with terrible dysmenorrhoea (painful menstruation) and had special tablets from the GP. This was all very expensive and I had to arrange my off duty times to cover the first two days of menstruation. The routine was hot bath, hot drinks, hot water bottle and dysmen. tablets. Sex was very painful. I had a retroverted uterus, and used any excuse not to have sex.

'Four years ago, at work, I felt really ill. My period was about five days late. I started to be sick and the GP I was working with told me to rest while he carried on with the ante-natal clinic. I continued to be violently sick with abdominal tenderness. The doctor (also my own GP) sent me for admission to the gynaecology ward, as he thought I had an ectopic pregnancy. The next morning I had a scan, which showed two fibroids inside the uterus and one on the outside. I was in so much pain that I had fainted a few times.

'The consultant came to see me at midday and told me he would have to do a hysterectomy. I shook my head and began to shake with apprehension. He had an operation list that afternoon and would put me on the end. How did I feel about that? I asked for my husband, Matthew, who came up straight away and spoke to the consultant. Matthew felt there was something very seriously wrong and that the consultant was holding back, but said it would be the best thing for me because of my history of DVT. Matthew said the consultant was a good surgeon, whom I had worked with and who had delivered our second child. He felt I was in good hands and that the consultant would do everything possible for me. In

Jamaica there is a real stigma attached to hysterectomy; you are not a woman any more if you have one. This did not affect either my husband or myself. The fear of another DVT (I had now experienced two) and the need to be heparinised (injected with heparin to stop the clotting of the blood) was greater than any worry about hysterectomy.

'My reaction was: "Oh God, can I run away down the back stairs?" Palpitations, headache and nervous twitch got the better of me. I prayed that God would look after me, see me safely to theatre and back!! I could not collect my thoughts as to what I should be praying for. I would love to have had my minister or someone to pray for and with me. I opened my eyes and there was the chief phlebotanist (a specialist in blood clotting disorders) coming to see me. He had seen my name on a sample and come to see if it really was me. He is a Christian and an elder in his church (Methodist). I thought he was an angel stood there at my door, in his white coat. He prayed for me, asking God to give me the courage and strength to go forth with the operation, for faith and trust in the Lord that it would be successful and that my family would be very supportive and understanding. No sooner had he gone than my nurse manager came along. She said later that I looked grey, distant and very frightened and that she had to talk to me. What she said I don't know. The next person through the door was the Methodist minister, who also prayed with me. I felt the Lord was truly with me.

'The operation was successful. Later that week, the consultant told me and my husband, in front of the children (11 and 9 years old) that there was no cancer. My husband felt he could have been a bit more subtle, but I think he was so pleased to tell me the news that he was not conscious the children were there. I went home on the tenth day, feeling a little tired and with some pain only on movement. The family were glad to have me home again. My husband was very supportive and helpful, insisting that I sit down or go to bed and do nothing. The children tried their best not to upset me in any way.

'I have made an excellent recovery. I'm back in full-time employment and also run a very successful women's self-help group, HSG. Sex is good, I haven't had any pain since the op and no problems at all. I have asked my husband if he feels any difference, and he doesn't, but then things are so much better anyway.'

## CHRIS

Chris, married but childless, had an emergency total abdominal hysterectomy when 27, fourteen years ago. Problems started with her periods at 16. Bleeding was scanty, but her stomach would swell to the size of a six-month pregnancy. Two D and Cs made little difference, and the doctor said it would resolve after a pregnancy. Chris married at 20, but experienced two traumatic miscarriages in the first two years. While recovering from the second, her husband left her for her friend and she went back to live at home. Her mother became ill and Chris nursed her until she died, later that year. When Chris was 25 she met her second husband, Tony, but when she became pregnant two years later, lost that baby as well. Her younger sister was pregnant at the same time, but sadly had toxaemia and died in Chris's arms. Her baby died as well.

'All that year I was in and out of hospital to try and find out why I kept losing babies. Then I was rushed to hospital in severe pain. An ectopic (tubal) pregnancy was diagnosed and I had an emergency op. I don't remember much of the first few days post-op as I was given a drug, which I was allergic to and was very ill. When I finally came round enough to realize what was going on, I was getting hot flushes. The doctors had found such a mess, an ovarian cyst on one ovary, both tubes blocked from all the other operations, a pregnancy in one tube and a rather underdeveloped womb, the reason for all my miscarriages. They had decided enough was enough, and had taken the lot away! They had left a small part of one ovary, but said that I would have menopausal symptoms for ten years. I would never be able to have a baby! I don't remember the rest of my hospital stay, I suppose I was in a state of shock. I was 27 years old.

'When I got home, there was a song on the TV about being a nanny to hundreds, but mother to none. That's the time it really hit me that I would never have a baby of my own. I suppose that's the time I let it all come out and my husband sent for the doctor, who put me on Valium. I stayed on it for quite a long time. I remember there was a young woman who faked pregnancy and then took a baby. I really understood how she felt, because I felt just the same. I went through about six months when I could have taken a baby and not given the mother a second thought. Then I had another couple of months when I could have killed any baby I saw. These emotions were so strong that they really upset me and I felt that I just wanted to die. I couldn't see any way out of the deep anger, resentment and loneliness that lay ahead of me for the rest of my life. All I had ever wanted was to be married and have kids and be happy. Tony just couldn't understand the deep need I had for a baby and our marriage just fell apart. I was now nearly eleven stone and couldn't care less about anything.

'I went to the doctor for something for the menopausal feelings I'd had since the op. He said that as I was still young and sexually active, that would be all I needed, to go away, lose weight and get on with life! So I took a good look at myself in the mirror and didn't like what I saw. I decided to go on a diet, get back into nursing and take my finals. I left Tony, got down to forty-eight kilograms (eight stone) and passed my nursing finals.

'When I met Michael I found it very difficult to let him get close and it took a long time before I really got involved with him. His mum and dad didn't want us to get married because there would be no grandchildren. Michael didn't see this as a problem and he accepted the fact that there would be no children. We did try to adopt, but didn't go through with it. I would love to have Michael's baby and it upsets me that I can't. Our relationship is very close, and I would be a very possessive mum, so it would probably come between us. It doesn't stop the longing when I hold a new baby or the resentment that I had the choice taken away.

'I have a different doctor now, but he won't prescribe HRT either. A couple of years ago, the menopausal problems increased, with the flushes, night sweats, and sleeplessness getting worse. I lost concentration and memory, and started panic attacks, aches in all my joints and, the most upsetting of all, periods of blankness, even when driving. The woman doctor at the Well Women Clinic said that I am menopausal, but she cannot give me HRT without my doctor's consent. Where do I go from here? I hurt my wrist by just pulling on the hand brake in the car and it was strapped up in Casualty. The doctor thought there was misplacement of bones. Could I be starting osteoporosis? It was really too soon to tell, he said. I carry on with what I am doing for myself with calcium tablets, cod liver oil, Vit B6 and now Evening Primrose Oil to see if that helps.

'As far as I'm concerned, having a hysterectomy was one of the worst things that ever happened to me. I didn't even have the choice. It has been difficult to put down into words all the pain and hurt that I have felt over these years. Reading this through I thought "Poor thing". I felt as if it had happened to someone else.'


## MRS MANN

Mrs Mann, widowed with two married children, had an emergency total abdominal hysterectomy with removal of ovaries, at 62, two years ago. Mrs Mann had no previous health problems. At 54 she had started the change, which seemed to go well. Her husband, Bill, had a heart attack and died nine months before she had the op.

'I was devastated by Bill's death; it was all so sudden, I hardly noticed what was happening to myself. I remember odd twinges of pain in my right side. My ankles began to swell and my legs ached at times. I had looked so young for my age with a trim figure, but with Bill gone I just let things go and I put on weight. My children were worried, but I felt they had their own lives and families to look after. I tried to be cheerful when they visited, bottling up the loneliness and hurt. I felt out of sorts and miserable, a bit like a lost soul. When I began to feel sick at times I thought it was to do with something I had eaten, or not eaten! Sometimes I did forget to eat. Shortly after that I woke one night with the most awful pain in my stomach; I was sweating and vomiting. My GP came out quite quickly and after examining me, ordered me away to hospital.

'There they did all sorts of tests, put up a drip and gave me something strong by injection for the pain. The doctor said it was an emergency and that they would want to operate quickly. The consultant came with the results of the morning's tests and said they would operate that afternoon. I had an enlarged ovarian cyst that had caused all the trouble and it would have to come out. I was to have a hysterectomy! I can remember thinking, What a strange thing, my periods finished years ago. Surely he doesn't mean a hysterectomy. I'm too old for that kind of thing. I never even asked him about it, but of course he did mean a hysterectomy. The nurses and doctors looked after me so well and I went home on the tenth day.

'The hospital arranged for a home help and also convalescence for me two weeks later. At the post-op check, I was told the cyst showed signs of cancer, but they had got it in time and I wouldn't need further treatment. I was very lucky, as it had twisted round on itself and so gave a sign it was there.

'The family rallied round, but I found as I got better physically, I felt very tearful and sad. I hadn't ever been like this, even when Bill died, and I thought that this was the result of the hysterectomy. I felt so lonely, Bill and I had shared so much. We'd been married forty years and sometimes we didn't need words even to know what the other was thinking. I missed him so badly, and I needed him. I got pretty low and by chance spoke to someone about being depressed after my op. I ended up going to a bereavement counsellor and things began to slot into place. I was still grieving over Bill, the shock had numbed me for some months and then I tried to keep a stiff upper lip. People had expected me to be over Bill and in fact it seemed to get worse. Then, with the suddenness of the op and being so low afterwards, all the hurt, anger and even bitterness of that year welled up.

'The hysterectomy saved my life. I felt a freak having it at my age, but I've since met women older than me, one who was 80 when she had hers! I was very lucky I made a quick recovery and I do keep in touch with the hospital with a regular check-up. Sex isn't important without Bill.'

# 10.
# PROLAPSE

Sometimes, the supports of the womb can be weakened,
for example, during childbirth, and the vaginal/rectal
(back passage) and vaginal/urethral (front passage) walls
become overstretched. The resulting prolapse can be
slight, affecting only one vaginal wall, or extensive, with
the womb actually protruding out of the vagina. If the
surgery needed to repair this is extensive and/or the
woman doesn't want any more children, or is over 35, a
hysterectomy may be performed at the same time as the
repair. This may mean the removal of a healthy womb,
but is seen as effecting a better repair and forestalling
further problems. Symptoms can vary from slight
discomfort to heavy bleeding and pain with restriction of
movement at certain times of the month, and urinary and
bowel problems.

Three of the women in this chapter had a vaginal
hysterectomy and repair; two were childless. The ages
range from 42 to 74.

## KITTY

Married with two adult children, Kitty had a vaginal
hysterectomy and repair at 48, seven years ago.

'My problems began with the birth of my daughter,
when I was 25. I was told that "things" had not
gone back properly, but not to worry. I went to my GP
many times over the years, but was told: "All's okay." My
periods were heavy and painful and I had backache. My
sex life was an anxiety, not an enjoyment, but none of this
mattered at all. The birth of my second baby hadn't
helped the situation, either.

'I decided seven years ago that a visit to my new GP was

vital, and when he diagnosed a prolapse, my only emotion was *joy*. Yes joy, after all those years, not good years by any stretch of the imagination. I was not surprised when told I needed a vaginal hysterectomy. It also proved to my husband that I had not been "faking" difficulties and pain simply to get out of loving him. I had gleaned information about hysterectomy from other women who I'd worked with, who'd had the op. Mine was slightly different in that it was to be vaginal and I would have no outward scars. I wanted to get it over so I could get on with my life.

'My stay in hospital was quite pleasant with nurses, doctors and fellow patients very friendly and helpful. They don't tell you a lot and I still don't know very much about how the op is performed or anything like that. It was not a bad experience and certainly nothing to be afraid of. I was away from work for eight weeks and when I went back I felt like a different person. I didn't have to count up "my time" and could go out without taking supplies. I felt more feminine somehow, at last I could really love my husband. We almost had a second honeymoon, only it was better than the first time.

'I can look back on my op as the opening of a door on to a more carefree and active way of life. I had made a full, fast recovery and wondered what all the fuss was about. Two years later I began to think something else was wrong, but how could it be? I had nothing left "downstairs". The diagnosis was ovarian cysts and I had to have both ovaries removed. That is a different story, and took many years to get over! But only good came out of my hysterectomy; it was one of the best things that has happened to me.'

## MIRIAM

Miriam, married with two teenage sons, had a vaginal hysterectomy and repair at 42, eight years ago. Miriam had long-term problems with very bad, heavy, painful periods. These worsened when she came off the pill, aged 39, and she received a variety of treatments from her GP to no avail.

'My GP, a fantastic man, referred me to a gynaecologist, who I saw privately. He examined me and said I had a very enlarged womb which had prolapsed, causing the pains and discomfort, and advised a hysterectomy. I was flabbergasted, the news devastated me. I thought it was an older woman's operation, not what I needed. I didn't know anyone who'd had it, and I'd never heard of a *vaginal* hysterectomy. When asked if there was another way I could be helped, he simply said, "Don't have it done, stay as you are!", which was very comforting!!

'I didn't know what hysterectomy meant, but found out and it didn't bother me. I was worried about having major surgery, as I'd never had an op before. I talked it over with my husband, and decided to go ahead. We didn't have any money to pay for the op and decided to wait on the NHS. My symptoms got a lot worse and I had to spend a couple of days each month in bed. Even on holiday! Then, at last, a letter came for admission to hospital!

'I was coward enough not to want to know anything before the op. I reacted badly to the anaesthetic and was very sick for a couple of days afterwards. I had a lot of discomfort and the morphine-based pain-killers didn't work for me. But the sister, unsympathetic at first, got the doctor to give me something weaker, but more effective. The other lady having the same surgery as me didn't have these problems. The doctor explained how they had done the op and I was amazed. I was thrilled to bits not to have a mark or blemish on my body. I am quite slim and was delighted to end up without a scar. He described my womb as very enlarged, but healthy, no cancer, and said the op had gone well with no problems. I was absolutely amazed to be told I would be discharged home after two days! I didn't feel ready and asked what to expect, but the nurses didn't know. There was no constructive advice, or leaflets. I refused to go home and stayed one more day!

'The consultant came round and saw us that night and told us: "There are no limitations now you've had the op done. Off you go and lead a normal life." I asked about taking things easy and he assured me it wasn't necessary. I thought he knew what he was talking about. I assumed that because of the way it's done, I could go home and everything would be fine. Walking warily, sitting gingerly, there was some discomfort but not much.

'Two days later I went off to support the football club we run at a match! I nearly passed out and was absolutely shattered. I had severe spasms of pain which continued the next day. I had a bath and began to lose fresh, red blood, where up to this time I hadn't had any loss post-op. This worried me, but the pains stopped. I saw the GP the next day, who said that the blood had congealed, causing a blockage and pain, and the bath had freed it. He didn't know how to advise me not having come across this type of op before. He didn't agree with the consultant and said I should take things easy, as I'd had major surgery. I should be guided by my instincts and rest, not overdo things, keep to light housework.

'I would just sit there and burst into tears, which worried me. I didn't realize it was a reaction to the operation and the loss of female organs. I felt like Jekyll and Hyde and worried about the personality change I was undergoing. My husband didn't know what was happening and we were both in the dark, but at least, together. I am lucky to have such an understanding husband. With a vaginal hysterectomy, nothing shows, it's all internal. Some men would expect wives to be back to normal immediately.

'My husband and sons were very supportive and it was lovely to have their total support. I think women need counselling, not because it's a terrible op, but because we need help through this time. Women should question having the op if they're not happy; they should be sure in their own minds. It's a good op if done for the right reasons, but some don't look into it too deeply and then afterwards regret it.

'I saw the consultant at the post-op check and said it was confusing that no one was giving answers, we just had to go through it to find out. Also that I was unhappy there wasn't information in hospital. He wasn't pleased and felt that women over-emphasized and made a meal of hysterectomy. He did "hundreds of operations" and knew what he was talking about! A typical chauvinistic attitude, I corrected him, that no matter how many he did, he knew nothing as he hadn't had one! He wasn't keen on any information leaflet.

'It would have been nice to talk to someone who'd been through it, instead of hearing all the old wives' tales. Your stomach falls out, you get very hairy, grow manly, your sex life goes!! I needed to talk to someone in those early days, when my stomach was still distended. I was fortunate that I'd kept in touch with the woman I was in hospital with, and also become involved with a women's self-help group, HSG. This has proved to be a much-needed service for others.

'I didn't feel like sex post-op, I was quite terrified it would make a difference. In fact, sex is very good and greatly improved. I no longer have the discomfort of monthly periods and I am the new woman they promised!'

## MIA

Mia, married and childless, had a vaginal hysterectomy and repair at 59, two years ago. Mia worked full time as a kitchen-hand on school meals.

'I had a lot of problems, not just pain, but leaking urine when I coughed or moved the tables at work. When the consultant said surgery could be done to correct this, I was surprised when he said hysterectomy. I thought of that as an op for younger women with period problems. I no longer had periods, but he said it was best to remove the womb, and I agreed.

'Following the op I went home and did no heavy housework at all. No hoovering, lifting or anything strenuous. I didn't drive or do the shopping until after my six-week check. Then I gradually started to get back into my usual routine and returned to work at ten weeks post-op. I did feel tired for a while, but on the whole everything seemed to be all right.

'I retired the following year and began to realize that all was *not* right. I felt as if something "down below" had dropped. I went back to the hospital and was taken in for a further vaginal repair. I was told this was needed as my muscles had stretched and that this was a problem of getting old.

'I rested for a couple of weeks afterwards and did not lift *anything*, generally taking things easy until three months post-op. So far I haven't had a recurrence and I feel quite different, even at this stage, from the first time round, better and more comfortable. The hysterectomy was not a problem in any way. My husband and I are very close, we do many things together, walking, hobbies and dancing. We share the housework, he has been retired five years and is good at cooking. Sex, as such, finished between us a few years back, so that remains unchanged.'

## NANCY

Nancy, single and childless, had an abdominal hysterectomy and vaginal repair four years ago, aged 74.

'My problems were mainly to do with a dropping of my womb, that pulled on the wall of the bladder and I kept getting bladder infections. I'd had these a long time, but my GP had said I was too old to have anything done. Later, he retired and the new man sent me to hospital. It was quite straightforward. The consultant said a hysterectomy and repair would help me and I said: "Thank you."

'I had no worries about having surgery or an anaesthetic. I felt it had to be done as I had so much I wanted to do and the constant visits to the doctor had been tiresome. My younger relatives were surprised that, at my age, I was having the op, and for prolapse problems, being childless. I discussed this with my new GP and he said age and family factors played a part. He also said I would make a quicker recovery than younger women, because of being past the change.

'I did recover quickly and went to stay with family for six weeks. I found it very frustrating not to do the usual things and hard to keep myself from getting bored. Once home, the most difficult things, I found, were getting the wet washing out of the machine and carrying shopping up the four flights of stairs to my flat. These were sorted out as I got stronger. Although I was pleased to be home for the quietness, I did appreciate staying with the family in the early days. I think being on one's own in those first few weeks, when you can't do much, could be very lonely and depressing.

'I have felt extremely well since and have been able to do the things I wanted. It is all now very much in the past and I hardly give it a thought.'

# 11.
# THE LAST MYTH

The last myth of hysterectomy is that women don't want to know, or even shouldn't be allowed to know, what is involved. It is felt that knowing about the negative as well as the positive side will worry women unnecessarily. They just don't cope well, or will make a poor recovery simply because they know of possible complications. Women are thought to imagine themselves into all sorts of physical and neurotic disorders. In many of the case studies, women not only wanted more information, but also wanted to be treated as partners and equals in the health choices facing them. One woman made an excellent recovery despite lack of information, but she felt her family didn't do so well. They paid a high price that was avoidable, because information hadn't been available. In fact, pre-op information and preparation enable women and their families to adjust to the surgery involved and plan for the recovery time. To know that wound, bladder, pelvic infections, bowel disturbances, lethargy or sadness can occur following hysterectomy is not to say they will, nor that the long-term effect of the operation is any less positive or desirable. We are all aware of how much physical exhaustion, or low physical reserves, affect emotional stability and ability to think logically. Yet, the fact that low-key chronic or recurring infections following on from major surgery (hysterectomy) might have the same effect, seems to have been ignored. Some women in this group were given unrealistic goals with too little information, not knowing what to expect, or how to cope with small, but chronic post-op difficulties. This did more to damage morale and prolong energy-sapping stressful emotions than anything else. Fortunately, this was often balanced by good social support from partners, close friends or women's support groups.

As one woman said, counselling is needed at this time, not that hysterectomy is a terrible experience, but because women need help through it. So what can women do to help themselves? No hysterectomy is an expected event in life, but we could become more aware of ourselves and value our health in a positive way. We can take note of symptoms that occur and go to the doctor. We can put ourselves in a position of value, and not delay because of family, job or other commitments, effectively putting our health needs last. We can ask what different treatments are available, why this one is tried first, what the side effects of the pills are; also, how long before they take effect, and what would follow on if they didn't work? If there seems to be delay, as in several of the case studies, then we can seek referral to a consultant. If the doctor has referred to a consultant, then we can check with the doctor as to what he expects the consultant to do – whether tests, a D and C or whatever. If the consultant suggests something different, we can then ask, why.

Confronting our own frailty is difficult, especially in situations that we barely know exist, and questioning takes us out of the passive state of accepting what 'fate' has to offer and puts us into a position of decision and responsibility. It can be an uncomfortable, insecure feeling when the final decision for hysterectomy is seen to be ours. For this we need the support of the doctor, amongst others, and adequate information. We need to know ourselves and what we can cope with in the way of symptoms and incapacity, what the threat to life, or the quality of life may be, pre-op as well as post-op. The risks against the gains! It's how we spend most of our life, balancing out the risks. We do it several times a day when crossing the road without a second thought, yet many thousands are maimed each year and several hundreds die on the roads. We don't stand dithering on the curb, weighed down by the fear of what we know might happen. We take all due care in the light of the knowledge available and make a decision on that. Hysterectomy is the same.

True, we can only have it out once and once gone, it's gone
for ever, but all the more reason to prepare well.

Find out the reason for the hysterectomy. Is it seen as a
'cure' for this, or part of continuing treatment? What sort
of hysterectomy is it to be? What is to be removed? Will
the ovaries be left? If not, what is the policy on HRT?
Would it be suitable in this case? Find out as much as
possible about hysterectomy, talk it over with family,
partner or close friend and explore what it means to you.
Make an effort to be physically fit: give up smoking, go for
daily walks, eat balanced, regular meals, check if any
medication prescribed should be stopped.

Doing these things does not mean that all will go in the
perfect text book way. As we saw from the case studies,
many factors influence reaction to, and recovery from,
hysterectomy. Post-op recovery, with or without
infections, is handled better by a body defence system in
peak condition. Mental and emotional preparation for this
time helps with the delays and frustrations that life can
toss up in the most unexpected manner at our most
vulnerable times, even if it means understanding that
some emotional issues need to be put off and faced at a
later date, so that precious reserves are channelled into
recovery.

It is true that the doctor and consultant are the experts,
but they are dependent on what we reveal to them of
ourselves and symptoms. We have lived a while with our
bodies and will have a gut reaction about suggested
treatments. It may be one of instant accord in recognition
that this is exactly right. It may be one of instant rejection
of advice either to have or not have a hysterectomy. It
may be dismay and numbness. Whatever the reaction,
take time to talk it out and adjust. Remember everyone is
an individual. If there is doubt about the reasons given, or
the need expressed, for or against hysterectomy, then
discuss this with the consultant, or get a second opinion
from another consultant. Do this by asking the GP to refer
to another gynaecologist at another hospital.

Write queries down, or take a friend for moral support. Plan for the recovery period at home, make arrangements with the GP and/or Social Services for heavy family commitments. This includes elderly relatives as well as children. Stock up the cupboard, freezer, and favours owed by friends, ready to call in after the op. Look at the possibility of convalescence, either through the GP, hospital social worker, or any union/professional representative on what is available and the cost.

A planned hysterectomy has so many advantages, allowing preparation of self, of family, job and domestic commitments. The trauma of an emergency carries a high price, despite being life-saving, and any who've had the experience would wish it had been different. Use of information and support resources within the statutory services and the voluntary sector can fill in many gaps of provision of support for women undergoing hysterectomy. Use of these also stimulates a better service for those yet to need it, as well as meeting something of the present demand.

Perhaps the most important thing is for every woman to be in tune with her own body and to follow what it indicates.

# USEFUL ADDRESSES

Many of the following have local therapists or groups. Ring for lists and information on services provided and possible charges.

Action for the Victims of Medical Accidents (AVMA)
01 291 2793
Advises patients who've been subjects of medical accidents. Can refer to medical experts for independent opinions.

Amarant Trust
14 Lord North Street
London SW1P 3LD
Gives information on how to get hormone replacement therapy.

Association of Community Health Councils for England and Wales
01 272 5459/5450
Each health authority has a CHC to represent the consumer of the NHS and will help with advice on services available in the area and in formulating letters to hospital administrators. Contact the above for local CHC.

Back Pain Association
31–3 Park Road
Teddington
Middlesex TW11 0AB
01 977 5474/5

Breast Care and Mastectomy Association of Great Britain
26 Harrison Street
Kings Cross
London WC1H 8JG
01 837 0908

British Acupuncture Association and Register
34 Aldernay Street
London SW1V 4EU
01 834 1012/3353

British Association for Counselling
37a Sheep Street
Rugby
Warwickshire CV21 3BX
078 78328/9
Information on local counsellors and also psychosexual
counselling.

British Association of Cancer United Patients (BACUP)
121–3 Charterhouse Street
London EC1M 6AA
01 608 1785
Provides leaflets on different types of cancer, including
those of the cervix, ovary and womb, and their treatments.
Telephone counselling and information service.

British Association of Psychotherapists
c/o 121 Hendon Lane
London N3 3PR
01 346 1747

British Chiropractors' Association
5 First Avenue
Chelmsford
Essex CM1 1RX
0245 358487

British College of Naturopathy and Osteopathy
Frazer House
6 Netherall Gardens
London NW3 5RR
01 435 8728
Provides treatment, self referral by ringing for price and appointment.

British Deaf Association
38 Victoria Place
Carlisle CA1 1HU
0228 48844

British Diabetic Association
10 Queen Anne Street
London W1M 0BD
01 323 1531

British Digestive Foundation
7 Chandos Street
Cavendish Square
London W1A 2LN
01 580 1155

British Epilepsy Association
Crowthorne House
Bigshotte
New Wokingham Road
Wokingham
Berkshire RG11 3AY
0344 773122

British Herbal Medicine Association
3 Amberwood House
Walkford
Christchurch
Dorset BH23 5RT
0202 431901

British Holistic Medical Association
179 Gloucester Place
London NW1 6DX
01 262 5299
List of medically qualified practitioners and literature.

British Homeopathic Association
27a Devonshire Street
London W1N 1RJ
01 935 2163
List of medically qualified practitioners.

British Osteopathic Association
8–10 Boston Place
London NW1 6QH
01 262 5250/1128
List of practitioners.

Cancer After-Care and Rehabilitation Society (CARE)
Lodge Cottage
Church Lane
Timsbury
Bath BA3 1LF
0761 70731
Moral support and advice.

Cancer Help Centre
Grove House
Cornwallis Grove
Clifton
Bristol BS8 4PG
0272 743216
Holistic healing, ring for fees and information on courses.

Cancer Link
46a Pentonville Road
London N1 9HF
01 833 2451
Provides information and support.

Cancer Relief
Macmillan Fund
Anchor House
15–19 Britten Street
London SW3 3TY
Nursing services at home and short stay nursing homes for cancer patients. Apply through a hospital social worker, district nurse, GP.

College of Health
18 Victoria Park Square
London E2 9PF
01 980 6263
Seeks to promote positive health through improved self care, use of NHS and alternative medicine. Healthline telephone information service.

Compassionate Friends
6 Denmark Street
Bristol BS1 5DQ
Bereavement support for stillbirth/death of baby, has local branches.

Council for Complementary and Alternative Medicine
Suite 1
19a Cavendish Square
London W1M 9AD
General council for alternative medicine therapies.

Cruse
Cruse House
126 Sheen Road
Richmond
Surrey TW9 1UR
01 940 4818
For bereavement support.

Depressives Anonymous
36 Chestnut Avenue
Beverley
North Humberside HU17 9QU

Depressives Associated
PO Box 5
Castletown
Portland
Dorset DT5 1BQ
Has penfriend scheme.

Dr Edward Bach Centre
Mount Vernon
Sotwell
Wallingford
Oxfordshire OX10 0PZ
Natural healing through wild flowers.

Drugs, Alcohol, Women, Nationally (DAWN)
Boundary House
91–3 Charterhouse Street
London EC1M 6HR
01 250 3284
Information, London area only.

Endometriosis Society
65 Holmdene Avenue
London SE24 9LD
01 737 4764, evenings.

Family Planning Association
FPA St Andrew's House
27–35 Mortimer Street
London W1N 7RJ
01 636 7866
Some clinics for Well Women and sexual difficulties.

Gingerbread
35 Wellington Street
London WC2E 7BN
01 240 0953
For one parent families.

Greek Cypriot Women's Health Group
Cypriot Community Centre
Earlham Grove
Wood Green
London N22
01 881 7826
Health talks.

Guild of St Raphael
St Marylebone Parish Church
Marylebone Road
London NW1 5LT
01 935 7315
Agency for the Churches Council of Healing, Church of
England.

Health Education Council
78 New Oxford Street
London WC1A 1AH
01 631 0930
Information leaflets on health topics.

Healthrights
157 Waterloo Road
London SE1 8XS
To improve individuals' and community rights in health
care. Advice on women's health, access to medical records
and medical ombudsman.

Herpes Association
41 North Road
London N7 9DP
01 609 9061

Holiday Care Service
2 Old Bank Chambers
Horley
Surrey RH6 9HW
02937 74535
Free service for elderly, disabled, single parents and those
with low income on appropriate holidays.

Hospice Information Service
St Christopher's Hospice
51–9 Lawrie Park Road
Sydenham
London SE26 6DZ
01 778 9252
Information about hospice units and teams for terminally
ill.

Hysterectomy Support Group
Moral support and information, pre- and post-op. Local
contacts. For booklet on preparation for post-op recovery
period, membership newsletters:
HSG c/o 11 Henryson Road
Brockley
London SE4 1HL
01 690 5987
General enquiries and local contact:
c/o WHRRIC
52 Featherstone Street
London EC1Y 8RT
01 251 6332

Institute of Marital Studies
Tavistock Centre
Belsize Lane
London NW3 5BA
01 435 7111
For marriage or sexual problems.

Intractable Pain Society of Great Britain and Ireland
Basingstoke District Hospital
Aldermaston Road
Basingstoke
Hampshire RG24 9NA
0256 473202 ext. 3453
For details of local pain clinics and centres.

Jewish Marriage Council
23 Ravenshurst Avenue
London NW4 4EL
01 203 6311
Deals with all relationship problems.

London Bereavement Projects Co-ordinating Group
c/o 68 Chalton Street
London NW1 1HY
Counselling for the bereaved.

Marie Curie Memorial Foundation
28 Belgrave Square
London SW1X 8QG
01 235 3325
Nursing care and homes for cancer patients.

Marie Stopes House
The Well Woman Centre
108 Whitfield Street
London W1P 6BE
01 388 0662
Telephone information and advice service on women's
health. Charge made for medical examinations.

National Association for Mental Health (MIND)
22 Harley Street
London W1
01 637 0741
Local branch in telephone book.

National Association for Pre-menstrual Syndrome
(NAPS)
25 Market Street
Guildford
Surrey GU1 4LB
0483 572715

National Marriage Guidance Council (RELATE)
Counselling for all relationships with some psychosexual
sessions. See telephone directory for nearest branch.

National Organisation for the Widowed (CRUSE)
Cruse House
126 Sheen Road
Richmond
Surrey TW9 1UR
01 940 4818/9047
Counselling service for the bereaved.

National Osteoporosis Society
PO Box 10
Barton Meade House
Radstock
Bath BA3 3YB
SAE for information about osteoporosis, prevention and
treatment.

Patients' Association
Room 33
18 Charing Cross Road
London WC2H 0HR
01 240 0671
Advises on complaints procedure, campaigns for right of
patients to see records, and confidentiality.

Pelvic Inflammatory Disease Group
c/o WHRRIC
52 Featherstone Street
London EC1Y 8RT
01 251 6332

Positive Health Centre for Autogenic Training
101 Harley Street
London W1N 1DF
01 935 1811
Provides training and also local autogenic tutors. Ring for
charges.

Premenstrual Syndrome Society
c/o The Secretary
Premsoc
PO Box 102
London SE1 7ES
Information on variety of approaches to PMS.

Pre-menstrual Tension Advisory Service
PO Box 268
Brighton
East Sussex BN3 1RW
0273 771366
Postal service using nutritional assessment and correction
to treat PMS. Ring for charges.

Samaritans
17 Uxbridge Road
Slough
Berkshire SL1 1SN
Offer support to those who feel suicidal. Local branch in
telephone directory.

Terrence Higgins Trust
BM AIDS
London WC1N 3XX
01 833 2971
Leaflets on AIDS. Telephone information and advice
service.

Women's Health and Reproductive Rights Information
Centre (WHRRIC)
52 Featherstone Street
London EC1Y 8RT
01 251 6580
Monday, Wednesday, Thursday, Friday 11am–5pm
All areas of women's health.

Women's Health Concern
17 Earls Terrace
London W8 6LP
01 602 6669
Women's health including HRT.

Women's National Cancer Control Campaign
1 South Audley Street
London W1Y 5DQ
01 499 7532
Advice on breast and cervical cancer.

# FURTHER READING

*Hysterectomy*
L. Dennerstein, C. Wood, G. Burrows
Oxford University Press.

*Hysterectomy and Vaginal Repair*
S. Haslett and M. Jennings
Beaconsfield.

*Woman's Experience of Sex*
Sheila Kitzinger
Collins.

*Oestrogen*
Dr Lila Nachtigall
Arlington
On Hormone Replacement Therapy.

*No Change*
Wendy Cooper
Arrow
On Hormone Replacement Therapy.

*Life Change*
Dr Barbara Evans
Pan
On menopause.

*Once A Month*
Dr K. Dalton
Fontana
On Pre-menstrual Syndrome.

*Understanding Pre-menstrual Tension*
Dr M. Brush
Pan.

*Understanding Endometriosis*
Caroline Hawkridge
Optima.

*Positive Smear*
Susan Quilliam
Penguin.

*Cervical Smear Test*
Albert Singer and Dr. Anne Szarewski
Optima.

*Brittle Bones and the Calcium Crisis*
Kathleen Mayes
Grapevine.

## CERVICAL SMEAR TEST
**What Every Woman Should Know**
Albert Singer FRCOG and Dr Anna Szarewski

Every woman who has ever been sexually active is at risk from cervical cancer, but it is a condition that can be prevented. This detailed illustrated guide explains what a cervical smear is, how it is done, and what it means if the result is positive, and deals with the emotional and psychological implications.
'. . . an excellent new book which should allay women's fears about cervical cancer testing.' **Daily Mirror**

0-356-15065-8                                              £5.99 (UK)


## UNDERSTANDING ENDOMETRIOSIS
Caroline Hawkridge

Written in conjunction with the Endometriosis Society, this book provides the most up-to-date and comprehensive information on the causes, diagnosis and treatment of this increasingly common gynaecological disorder.

0-356-15447-5                                              £5.99 (UK)


## THE MENOPAUSE
**Coping With The Change**
Dr Jean Coope

This invaluable guide answers frequently asked questions and provides practical advice on how to make the menopause a change for the better.

0-356-14511-1                                              £5.99 (UK)

## DIABETES AND PREGNANCY
Anna Knopfler

Diabetic mother Anna Knopfler provides clear information and reassurance on all aspects of diabetic management, pregnancy and childbirth.

0-356-15189-1      £5.99 (UK)


## AVOIDING OSTEOPOROSIS
Dr Allan Dixon and Dr Anthony Woolf

Osteoporosis causes pain and disability in one in four post-menopausal women; this practical guide examines causes and symptoms and outlines methods of prevention and treatment.

0-356-15445-9      £5.99 (UK)


## THE BREAST BOOK
John Cochrane MS, FRCS and Dr Anne Szarewski

Comprehensive information and advice on all aspects of breast health and care, including breastfeeding and breast cancer.

0-356-15416-5      £5.99 (UK)

## BELOW THE BELT
### A Woman's Guide To Genito-Urinary Infections
Denise Winn

This reassuring guide provides practical information on
the causes, symptoms and treatment of all the major
genital infections, ranging from thrush to AIDS.
'As some infections show few symptoms in women in the
early stages, but have serious consequences if left
untreated, this book is useful to refer to.' **City Limits**

0-356-12740-0                                    £5.99 (UK)


## SELF-HELP WITH PMS
### Escape from the Prison of Premenstrual Tension
Dr Michelle Harrison

A positive approach provides clear, up-to-date advice on
the problems of, and cures for, premenstrual syndrome.
'. . . a thought-provoking and valuable book on a little
understood subject.' **Health Visitor**
'. . . a lifeline for anyone trying to pull themselves out of
the misery of premenstrual tension.' **Guardian**

0-356-12559-9                                    £5.95 (UK)


## CYSTITIS
### A Woman Doctor's Guide to Prevention and Treatment
Dr Kathryn Schrotenboer with Sue Berkman

50% of women can expect to experience cystitis at some
time; designed to help women formulate their own
prevention plan, this book explains how to treat, and
perhaps even more importantly how to avoid, recurrent
attacks.

0-356-15448-3                                    £4.99 (UK)

## MENOPAUSE THE NATURAL WAY
### Dr Sadya Greenwood

Correcting myths and explaining all medical details, this comprehensive book answers all the questions that are asked about the menopause.

0-356-12561-0          £5.95 (UK)


## MISCARRIAGE
### Margaret Leroy

'clear, sensible information. . . . I would not hesitate to recommend it to anyone who wants to know more about miscarriage.' **Nursing Times**
'Anyone who has experienced a miscarriage should be directed to (this) book.' **The Lancet**

0-356-12888-1          £5.95 (UK)


## EXPERIENCES OF ABORTION
### Denise Winn

Interviews with women of different backgrounds present the first-hand experiences of coming to terms with the emotional aspects and consequences of having an abortion.

0-356-14140-3          £4.99 (UK)

## CAESAREAN BIRTH
### A Guide for Parents
Melissa Brooks with Dr Michael Rogers

This practical guide to all aspects of both planned and
emergancy caesarean birth shows how a caesarean can be
as positive an experience of birth as any other form of
delivery.

0-356-15847-0                                    £5.99 (UK)


## ALTERNATIVE MATERNITY
### Nicky Wesson

From acupuncture to cranial osteopathy to medical
herbalism, this book provides a comprehensive guide to
the range of alternative remedies and therapies available
for both mother and baby at all stages of maternity.
Covers conception, pregnancy, childbirth and early infant
care.

0-356-15412-2                                    £5.99 (UK)

All Optima books are available at your bookshop or newsagent, or can be ordered from the following address:

Optima, Cash Sales Department,
PO Box 11, Falmouth, Cornwall TR10 9EN

Please send cheque or postal order (no currency), and allow 60p for postage and packing for the first book, plus 25p for the second book and 15p for each additional book ordered up to a maximum charge of £1.90 in the UK.

Customers in Eire and BFPO please allow 60p for the first book, 25p for the second book plus 15p per copy for the next 7 books, thereafter 9p per book.

Overseas customers please allow £1.25 for postage and packing for the first book and 28p per copy for each additional book.

ANN WEBB has been involved in midwifery, district nursing and health visiting for over twenty years.

She helped to set up the Hysterectomy Support Group in 1980 with the aim of establishing an informal support network for women to share their experiences as they recovery from surgery.

*Experiences of Hysterectomy* is her first book, and reflects her commitment to the idea that women need accessible, accurate information in order to make informed decisions about hysterectomy.